T0098557

Advance Praise for
The Ultimate Cure for
Depression

"Finally! I can tell my patients there is a book that elaborates clearly on the bases we barely have the time to develop in our, oh so short, sessions. This is an intuitive and understandable paradigm for healing that is informative and concise and approaches the spiritual dimension of restoration that so many shy away from in an expert fashion. The fact that I work with Dr. Joy at the Crisis Response Center, and never fail to wonder at the calm and, yes, accepting joy that follows him into the room, should make my endorsement of his mindful book that much more meaningful."

Daniela Reid, M.D.
Board-Certified Psychiatrist,
Connections Health Solutions, Tucson, AZ

"It's a great honor to write this short piece for a man with a solid career. He is a man of integrity and impeccable character. This book speaks well of the deep love and compassion that he has for the wellbeing of his clients. I know him both personally and professionally and I can say that this book exemplifies his dedication and tenacity to find effective solutions for his patients' challenges. The book speaks well of his in-depth knowledge of mental health problems. His approach to solving these problems indicates that he has had multiple proven results. The book is a must-read for clinicians and patients alike. Very insightful!"

James Abanishe, MD
Board-Certified Psychiatrist & Owner, Mountain Dew
Behavioral Health, Tucson, AZ

"It is often the case that people in the helping professions take a reductionistic approach to caring for their patients, preferring to focus on specific aspects of behavior, experience, or just symptoms. In a very conversational tone Dr. Joy looks at the whole person in his new book. People tend to know about Maslow's hierarchy of needs, but many may not know he later put spirituality above self-actualization. This book's fresh exploration of emotional distress takes us from basic survival needs through need for social relationships and supports with a strong emphasis on faith, belief, and spirituality. It will be a welcome addition to most people's treasured books that are accessible and offer new insights each time you go back to them."

Mary Lou Graham, APRN, RN, LPC
Psychiatric and Mental Health Nurse Practitioner,
ML Therapies, LLC, New Britain, CT

"What a masterpiece! This is a life changing book authored by an expert with considerable experience on treating depression. It is a rope of hope for anyone drowning from depression and sunshine for anyone locked in the dark room of depression. In this book Dr. Joy explains how he has used the biopsychosocial model of depression to successfully develop a very powerful tool he has called Authentic Healing Process for Depression. It uses a multifaceted approach of self-efficacy, medications, and faith among others to effectively deal with the multifaceted nature of depression. This should be a standard text for all high school and college students and is a must-read for any leader in any field of endeavor. I thoroughly enjoyed reading it."

Bertha Serwa Ayi, MD, FACP, FIDSA, MBA
Infectious Disease Specialist, CEO & Medical Director,
Global Infectious Disease Services, PC, Potomac, MD
Pastor, International Central Gospel Church (ICGC) Jubilee
Temple, Baltimore, MD

"Most books that I have read on the subject matter of depression have a view of either faith or science. Dr. Joy Kwakuyi's book has married both the experience of faith and the knowledge of science in the pursuit of healing. It is a must-read for all health professionals and patients."

James M. Doe, MD
Internist, El Rio Health, Tucson, AZ

"It is enlightening to have a book that focuses on the spiritual aspect of managing depression. As mentioned in the book, treatment of mental health conditions and more specifically depression can never be complete without including the spiritual aspects. In America, many people tend to focus on medical and/ or therapy forms of treatment to manage mood problems. The description of how human beings are interconnected in three dimensions of body, soul, and spirit is key to managing depression. The reliance on the power of God to aid in the management of depression and anxiety can guide us to be more helpful clinicians to the patients that we serve. Thank you, Dr. Joy for highlighting the missing piece in the management of mental illnesses in our society."

Esther Kioko DNP, MSN, RN, PMHNP-BC
Owner of Tucson Behavioral Health Services, Tucson, AZ

"I feel privileged to be given the opportunity to say a few words about Dr. Joy Kwakuyi and his new book. Dr. Joy was one of my preceptors when I was in school to become a psychiatric nurse practitioner. My original plan was to precept with him for two weeks at most, but I ended up staying for a couple of months! Why? Because I was impressed by his calm nature in the midst of chaos, his confidence, knowledge of, and passion for psychiatry. His book, *The Ultimate Cure for Depression? Leveraging Science and Faith for Total Healing* written from the heart is captivating and provides an effective and practical approach to healing. If you are suffering with depression or any other mood disorder, consider this a gift, read, and follow the recommendations to guide, encourage, and liberate you from your suffering."

Fuanjia Fuangunyi, DNP, APRN, PMHNP-BC
Psychiatric and Mental Health Nurse Practitioner, Tucson AZ

"In this therapeutic book, Dr. Kwakuyi writes: 'There is a surprisingly large number of individuals who are afflicted with depression and anxiety. A significant portion of this population is in the upper-middle income bracket, namely politicians, pastors, celebrities, business executives, lawyers, and professionals of all walks of life. Depression destroys lives, steals joy, deflates passions and ultimately wipes away destinies. Unfortunately, many people fail to actively seek help promptly when they are depressed. This book is not just a set of treatment recommendations. It is a combination of most of what the scientific world and the spiritual world have to offer on overcoming depression.' As a pastor, marriage teacher and counselor for over three decades, I highly recommend this book. Please grab a copy for yourself and some more for other people you may know who need your support."

Rev. Dr. Frank Opoku-Amoako
Apostolic Overseer,
Kings Destiny International Churches,
Manassas Park, VA

"An awesome book for all. A must-read book! This book has tools that can bring comfort and healing to the distressed and emotional resilience to every reader. In fact, one does not have to be depressed to read this book!"

John Forson, Pharm D, RPh.
Founder & Pharmacist-In-Charge,
North Capitol Pharmacy, Washington DC
Pastor, International Central Gospel Church (ICGC)
Glory Temple, Sterling, VA

"Dr. Joy Kwakuyi's writing style is so easy to follow. In my view, this book is written for both individuals in the medical field and the general public. Dr. Kwakuyi describes his approach of addressing depression using The Authentic Healing Process for Depression. The Authentic Healing Process for Depression is based on five concepts: Self-efficacy, biochemistry, spirituality, social connections, and working with experts. The book focuses on each concept, clearly defines each concept, and provides practical methods that the reader can use in battling depression.

Dr. Kwakuyi, in the entire book, narrates numerous experiences he has encountered in the clinical setting to reinforce the points he made in the book. This captivates the attention of the reader and makes the book relatable. The narration of his experiences in clinical practice is unique and helps the reader develop an understanding, respect, and appreciation of the Authentic Healing Process for Depression. The book provides a common thread that helps unite people from different cultures, knowing you are not alone in the fight. This provides a bridge across cultural gaps.

I must say I was skeptical before I read the book mainly because as a provider, I was not sure how one would incorporate faith in the treatment of individuals in healthcare. Western medicine focuses mainly on medications and other therapies depending on the specialty. Incorporating faith-based healing was never brought to my attention before reading the book. The Authentic Healing Process for Depression is based on the biopsychosocial-spiritual model, which has been used in psychiatry and has proven to yield results. Dr. Kwakuyi describes in detail how to approach a patient in order to incorporate the spiritual component in the plan of care. The book also mentioned Christian

Cognitive Behavioral Therapy which can be incorporated into the plan of care and is an evidenced based intervention. All in all, the book was an eye opener on a different treatment model."

Stephen K. Karuga, DNP, FNP-BC
Family Nurse Practitioner, Tucson, AZ

"Depression and anxiety are among mental health disorders that need to be addressed through comprehensive strategies that empower people to consider treatment towards recovery and long-term mental health promotion and prevention behaviors.[1] Occasionally a book is written with focus and purpose that feels like it was written just for you. This is such a book written to encourage people from all walks of like to seek care for depression and for other emotional and mental health challenges afflicting them. The author, Dr. Joy carefully balanced his professional psychiatric nurse practitioner knowledge with his deep Christian faith, desires and experiences in this non-technical easy to read book. Dr Joy is also upfront by indicating that the work in the book is heartfelt, it is an expression of opinion and observations and certainly not based on lots of research information but is needed to break the bond of inaction.

The author must have 'seen it all' as a practicing psychiatric provider and as a Christian minister. Chapter one provides an enlightening introduction that guides the reader through the spectrum of emotions that people afflicted with depression can recognize and use to self-diagnose as the first step towards seeking care. The chapter reminds readers about the vicious nature of depression and encourages people to let go of perceptions and seek care. Chapter two is an exposition of the authors personal life. Even though this chapter covered the details of personal life events which acted like signposts leading to the writing of this book, I appreciate the courage of the author in laying bare all his family history including vulnerabilities. They show that the message in the book is not born out of privileges, but passion and it is about inspiring others to take the step and towards healing.

Chapter four to chapter eight present information on the multidimensional tool that the author developed and has been using to treat depression. The tool called the Authentic Healing Process for Depression (AHPD) is a great demonstration of how an integrated treatment approach could be implemented. The AHPD integrated approach combined biochemical, spiritual, social professional and self-centered dimensions which aim for long lasting treatment effect. The approach highlights the fact that depression may be caused by many factors and this may explain why fragmented treatment approaches may not deliver long-lasting remission from depression. However, there is flexibility. The book explains how professional assessments can be used to customize the AHPD for different people. The theme on flexibility was extended to chapter nine where the author provides options for using the information in the book. The chapter discusses the possibility of individuals embarking on the treatment journey alone but emphasize the importance of working with professionals (especially, biomedical professionals who also believe in the effectiveness of all the dimensions included in the AHPD). The book concludes with chapter ten with a summary and suggested activities for total healing from depression.

Although I enjoyed reading the whole book, I personally found the chapters on the individual domains of the integrated treatment tool interesting and empowering, due to their detailed and comprehensive nature. In summary, this book provides a rich personal and professional information that combines traditional treatment approach with faith-based therapy from a strategic point of view. The book will be a very useful resource for people who are struggling to come to terms with the sadness and desperation inflicted by depression. The Christian Cognitive Behavioral Therapy approach adopted in the book also added a unique flavor which may encourage people to explore treatment dimensions beyond traditional approaches.

Conflict of Interest: The author and this reviewer are first cousins."

Janet Dzator, Ph.D.
Health Economist; Senior Lecturer,
University of Newcastle, NSW, Australia.
World Health Organization (WHO). 2013. Mental Health
Action Plan 2013-2030, Geneva, Switzerland

The Ultimate Cure for Depression

THE
ULTIMATE
CURE
FOR
DEPRESSION

Leveraging SCIENCE and
FAITH for Total Healing

DR. JOY KWAKUYI

NEW YORK

LONDON • NASHVILLE • MELBOURNE • VANCOUVER

The Ultimate Cure for Depression

Leveraging Science and Faith for Total Healing

© 2020 Dr. Joy Kwakuyi

All rights reserved. No portion of this book may be reproduced, stored in a retrieval system, or transmitted in any form or by any means—electronic, mechanical, photocopy, recording, scanning, or other—except for brief quotations in critical reviews or articles, without the prior written permission of the publisher.

Published in New York, New York, by Morgan James Publishing in partnership with Difference Press. Morgan James is a trademark of Morgan James, LLC. www.MorganJamesPublishing.com

ISBN 9781642797718 paperback
ISBN 9781642797725 eBook
ISBN 9781642797732 audiobook
Library of Congress Control Number: 2019913214

Cover Design Concept:
Difference Press

Cover Design by:
Rachel Lopez
www.r2cdesign.com

Interior Design by:
Christopher Kirk
www.GFSstudio.com

Editor:
Cory Hott

Book Coaching:
The Author Incubator

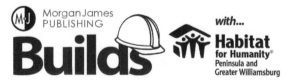

Morgan James is a proud partner of Habitat for Humanity Peninsula and Greater Williamsburg. Partners in building since 2006.

Get involved today! Visit
MorganJamesPublishing.com/giving-back

To the loves of my life: Esenam, Elsie, Ellis, and Elton.
To all who have suffered with depression.
You will overcome!

Table of Contents

Foreword

Depression is one of the most prevalent psychological giants of our age. Today, it is treated largely with medication and talk therapy. However, after many years of treating depression as a successful psychiatric nursing professional, the author of this book, Dr. Joy Kwakuyi, has discovered that adding the spiritual dimension to the recovery process improves results tremendously. Unfortunately, many Christians do not fully understand what the Bible teaches us about recovery from depression.

Students of the Bible have long known that the Bible is a veritable, unending source of revelation and that the scriptures contain the directions necessary for living a godly and victorious life. In 2 Timothy 3:16-17, we read, "All Scripture is given by inspiration of God, and is profitable for doctrine, for reproof, for correction, for instruction in righteousness, that the man of God may be complete, thoroughly equipped for every good work."

At the deepest level, the Bible provides symbolic and analogical clues to understanding spiritual and psychological truth in the Bible stories. The Bible itself says that this is true. According to 1 Corinthians 10:1, "Moreover, brethren, I do not want you to be unaware that all our fathers were under the cloud, all passed through the sea." In verse four of the same chapter, we read, "… and all drank the same spiritual drink. For they drank of that spiritual Rock that followed them, and that Rock was Christ." The Bible also tells us that these stories were written to provide truths that still apply today. 1 Corinthians 10:11, "Now all these things happened to them as examples, and they were written for our admonition, upon whom the ends of the ages have come."

As we search the Bible, the most detailed example of depression is included in the life of Elijah. Our story begins in 1 Kings Chapters 18-19.

Many times, depression follows periods of great accomplishment, failure, loss, or expenditure of energy. Elijah was a prophet of God during the reign of Ahab and Jezebel. Jezebel killed the prophets of God and promoted the fertility god, Baal. After a three-year famine, Elijah confronted Ahab and the prophets of Baal and proved to the people that Jehovah was God, by bringing down fire from heaven that consumed the sacrifice, stones and even the water around the altar. He killed four hundred prophets of Baal, prayed for rain (which resulted in a deluge), and out-raced Ahab's chariot back to Jezreel, the capital city. When Ahab told Jezebel what had happened, she sent a message threatening Elijah's life. He so feared Jezebel, that he ran for his life to Beersheba on the edge of Israel. Elijah took a day's journey into the wilderness and sat under a juniper tree which usually stands for "a defeated spirit, a disappointed life, and a depressed soul." In 1 Kings 18:4 Elijah says, "It is enough; now, O LORD, take away my life; for I [am] not better than my fathers." He had hoped that the great miracle of bringing down fire from heaven would turn the nation to God. In his eyes, he had failed.

In this book, Dr. Joy describes the treatment for depression as five domains or dimensions which correspond to the treatment process described in the Bible.

The Biomedical Dimension: This involves nourishment, sleep, physical exercise, and anti-depressants. While Elijah slept, an angel prepared a cake baked on coals for him to eat and gave him a container of water to drink. After sleeping and eating again, Elijah traveled forty days and nights to Mount Horeb, the site of most of God's Old Testament revelations to humanity. Studies have indicated that exercise can be as effective as anti-depression medication in alleviating mild to moderate depression.

The Spiritual Dimension: When Elijah got to a cave on the mountain, there was a great wind on the mountain that tore trees out by their roots, then an earthquake that broke rocks in pieces and, finally, a fire that devoured the mountain; but God was not in any of these. These events challenged Elijah's assumption that to have significant results, God would have to do spectacular things and He was out of options. Instead, God usually chooses to operate behind the scenes in almost undetectable ways. In this case, God spoke in a still, small voice to change Elijah's thinking. He still had a mission in life to accomplish and God would still make it happen. He just needed to hold onto his faith in God.

The Self-Efficacy Dimension: In the lowest moments of their lives, individuals that are depressed must be challenged to reevaluate their thinking and see their situations differently. When questioned, Elijah repeated his erroneous viewpoint, "I have been very jealous for the Lord God of hosts: for the children of Israel have forsaken thy covenant, thrown down thine altars, and slain thy prophets with the sword; and I, [even] I only, am left; and they seek my life, to take it away." (1 Kings 19:14) When depressed, we usually feel over-responsible in our situations and we need to recognize our true position in life. God revealed to Elijah that He still had seven thousand other people in Israel that had never worshipped Baal. (1 Kings 19:18) Elijah was not alone. God still had a plan for his life. Neither he nor God had failed and were out of options.

The Social Dimension: In pursuing a new vision for life, the person who is depressed must choose to act according to that direction and get out of isolation. Elijah called Elisha as the next prophet, and Elisha anointed new kings over Syria and Israel who overthrew Ahab and Jezebel, the very thing Elijah had failed to do. Restoration is complete when a person who was depressed again has the energy to invest in a renewed life and vision.

The Professional Dimension: Elijah was set free as he acted according to God's will and began to disciple Elisha. Elisha did twice as many miracles as Elijah had done. Although in Elijah's time they did not have psychiatrists, psychologists, therapists, and psychiatric nurse practitioners, with adequate knowledge and the application of the principles in this book, hopefully these professionals will also be able to provide "miracles" of deliverance from depression as God did for Elijah.

In this book, Dr. Joy provides a detailed and expansive understanding of how to integrate both biblical and medical principles in both self-help and clinical settings today.

Troy D. Reiner, PhD, LCMFT, LCAC
Director, Word of Life Counseling Center
& Word of Life Counseling Training Institute
Associate Pastor, Word of Life Church
Charter Member of the American
Association of Christian Counselors
Author of *Faith Therapy, Transformation,Revelations that Will Set you Free* and *Principles for Life*

Introduction

Welcome to a life-transforming journey!

When I started my outpatient psychiatric practice, Tucson Treatment Center, Inc., a few years ago, I quickly became overwhelmed by the large number of individuals who are afflicted with depression and anxiety. I was even more astonished when I discovered that a significant portion of this population are in the upper-middle income bracket, namely politicians, pastors, celebrities, business executives, lawyers, and professionals of all walks of life. This discovery is the underlying motivation for this project.

The average person desires to live a productive and fulfilling life. However, many things often rob us of this dream. One of these thieves is depression. Depression is a leading cause of disability in the world. Depression discolors lives, steals our joy, and deflates our passion. Depression wipes away destinies.

Unfortunately, all over the world, many people fail to intervene actively or seek help promptly when they are depressed. While this is true for many groups, one group of people who fail to seek help promptly are leaders in all spheres of life, including parents, community leaders, business leaders, church leaders, and other busy professionals. This is because they are expected to be strong so others can draw hope from them. We often forget that depression afflicts people from all walks of life. For this reason, depression has become an enemy so vicious and so deadly that we cannot afford to sit around passively and watch it destroy our lives or the lives of our loved ones.

This, and many other reasons, is why I wrote this book. I came to a point in my life when it became obvious that I had to write a book on depression. There were no two ways about it. I felt obligated. I must let out what is locked up within me. I am a firm believer in the fact that everyone came into this world fully loaded with virtue and potential. This endowment is meant to help to improve our world and the lives of others. Until we intentionally take steps to deliver or deploy these goods in some form, we will add to the wealth of the cemetery. I am therefore on a mission to ensure that I will eventually die empty, so to speak. Do join me in this journey.

As you will see, this book is part of my divine calling. My mother was not wrong when she chose my first name. As an individual, by default, I share joy and I teach joy. Because of this, many people have asked me over the years to package my teachings into a book. I am glad I could finally do so. Throughout my life, I have served as a source of encouragement and motivation for others. My life's journey brought me to a deep personal conviction that I am meant to be a channel of hope, purpose, and healing to my generation and beyond. Hopefully, by reading this book, you, my reader, will derive hope, purpose, and a new motivation for living a fulfilling life and soar above the many emotional challenges that you might face.

Additionally, I wrote this book because I meet people daily who I believe can use the information that I have included here. Everywhere I turn, I see someone hurting. The wounds are not always visible. I meet people every day who have lost interest in living and are only existing. This is probably because of the negative experiences and emotions that they have gone through and continue to go through in their lives. All too soon, you come to terms with the fact that life is not always as happy and bubbly as you desire, neither is life always fair. Many are successful in some areas of their lives, but they lack the joy of living because other areas of their lives are not working out as desired.

At my clinic, I wanted to develop a tool for teaching my patients. I ended up making a hand-written chart of all the interventions that help people to recover from their emotional and mental health challenges. Even today, I pull up this chart whenever I talk with my patients as a way of illustrating what they need to be doing. This chart highlights things like taking medications, attending appointments, developing and using coping skills, building and leveraging support systems, seeing a therapist, and improving sleep and appetite. I would often promise them that I would have the chart professionally designed whenever I get the opportunity. Later, I realized that a chart alone is not enough; a book is even better as it helps to explain all the aspects in more detail.

Traditionally, when people become depressed, we prescribe medications, and we provide talk therapy. Then, we advise them to sleep well, eat healthily, exercise often, and use positive coping skills—this is the most we do. Usually, only medications and therapy are recommended. Hence, we often fail to obtain effective and lasting results. No wonder many patients return to the psychiatric office so often with the news that they are still depressed despite the interventions. This is one of my motivations for writing this book: I discovered and wanted to propose a set of interventions that is more effective than the traditional interventions for depression.

This book is not just a set of treatment recommendations. It is an embodiment of my life, lived out, tested, and proven. It is what I believe in, and I hope you do, too. It is a combination of most of what the scientific world and the spiritual world have to offer on overcoming depression. It is my understanding and interpretation of what constitutes best practices for living a joy-filled and fulfilled life. It is a life packaged into a book. It is me combining what I do—mental health care and Christian ministry—into effective interventions for a life worth living.

Our lives extend beyond our time on earth. If you follow the lessons in this book, you will quickly realize that you have not only found a solution to depression, but you have a solution to life itself. You will realize that you not only live a fulfilled life on the earth, but you will also have a tangible hope for your future and a confidence that you will spend eternity with God. The truth is life does continue, even after death!

In this book, I use the word depression in a broad sense to represent a group of low moods, despair, despondency, and difficulty experiencing joy. Although this book will have some value for the academic and clinical communities, I wrote this book specifically for the non-clinical person who is afflicted with depression and is searching for an authentic solution. However, this book goes beyond a treatment for depression. It is a life companion for anyone who has ever experienced sadness in life and anyone who is looking for the key to a fulfilled life. I wrote this book from my heart, not just from my mind and certainly not from lots and lots of research data. Finally, I wrote this book because I believe in you! I know that there is hope for your future. With some help and guidance, you will make it. Read on!

Safety First!

This book is a non-emergency life-long companion. If you have thoughts of suicide or causing harm to yourself or others, I highly recommend calling 911 or another crisis line in your locality, or speaking to a medical professional, a spiritual leader, or a community leader as a matter of urgency.

Chapter 1

Living in a Dark Place

"Here is the tragedy: When you are the victim of depression, not only do you feel utterly helpless and abandoned by the world, you also know that very few people can understand, or even begin to believe, that life can be this painful."
– Giles Andreae

Think about this for a moment: You are the only one who truly knows what you are going through in your life. Others may see or hear about what you are going through, but no one will have a first-hand appreciation of your deepest emotions. You know that you could be truly joyful. You know that you could be truly satisfied and fulfilled in life. You know that you could be living a truly meaningful life. But you are not. Is it your fault? Probably not. Just like the average person, you dreamed of building a truly happy life. Not only that but you also worked hard and pursued your dreams to some extent.

For all intents and purposes, you may have achieved some success in your endeavors. You might be successful as a professional in your chosen career. Many others look up to you. You may have a beautiful family. Your neighbors and friends consider you and your spouse a perfect couple. You may even be known as a good Christian. You try to be friendly, and you are generous with your smiles in public. Of course, whenever you are asked, "How are you?" You respond, "I am fine. Thank you." You say this because that is what our society expects from us. That is the norm. Here comes the million-dollar question. Read it slowly; then pause and think before answering, "Are—you—really—fine?"

You're Not Alone

If your answer to the above question was anything less than, "Yes, of course," I would like you to know that you are not alone. Of course, "not fine" can mean many different things. However, if your response means that you have any form of depressed mood or low emotional state, I would like you to know that you belong to a large group of people worldwide who share similar responses. Depression is more common than we like to admit. About 300 million people suffer from depression across the world. Depression is a major contributor to the global burden of disease and is considered as a leading cause of disability worldwide.[2] In the United States, 17.3 million adults, representing

7.1 percent of the adult population, have had at least one major depressive episode in the year 2017 alone.[3]

There are many kinds of depression. Depression falls on a wide spectrum starting from just feeling down as a result of an adverse event all the way through to having a severe, recurring major depressive disorder. What is more, depression is not a respecter of persons. Both great and small, wealthy and poor, religious and atheist fall victim to depression year after year. Again, you are not alone. Several others are walking this road right now as you read this.

How Bad Is It?

If you are like most people, you have been dealing with depression for a while. You might have become acquainted with sadness. You cry yourself to sleep. You say to yourself, "I don't know happiness." You tried to just get used to it, but it is rather hard to get used to. You tried multiple remedies on your own, sought help from several professionals, and followed their recommendations. You took several antidepressants over the years. You went to therapy. You cannot sleep no matter how hard you try. You took sleeping pills with little benefit. Maybe you belong to the other group of people who oversleep and cannot get out of bed.

You meet your best friend over coffee. It is a safe environment. You lament, "My life sucks! Despite my career success, I feel empty. I doubt if there is any such thing as true joy. Nothing brings me joy." You continue, "People think I am a happy person, but they are mistaken. What they don't know is that I put on fake smiles. I don't even know why I am still alive. I wish I can end it all, but I am too chicken." You quickly assure your friend, "Don't get me wrong. I will never do anything to myself, but I have virtually no interest in living." She tries to make some recommendations, but you interject, "Listen, I have tried everything—medications, meditation, yoga, exercise, therapy, et cetera, but I can't seem to get out of this dark place. Nothing works!"

Behind those broad smiles lies a deep, dark hole of persistent sadness that sticks to you and never lets go. A deep ugly hole of emotional pain lies beneath the facade. It is broad daylight, but in your private world, it is a dark, dark place. It is as if there is a dark cloud hanging over your head. You say to yourself, "I am worried that I will never get better. I am afraid that things will only go downhill from here."

Grave, But Not Beyond Repair

In the spring of 2018, a middle-aged woman called my office and made an appointment to see me for an evaluation. Let's call her Paula. She found my practice profile via online research and noticed that several of my patients had left positive reviews from their interactions with me. She was also drawn to me because she noticed that I am a Christian minister and she wanted to explore all available resources, including her faith, in resolving her problems. She is a senior law enforcement officer who received several awards for her outstanding work in her city. As you can imagine, Paula is a role model for many.

In her private life, Paula is divorced, the mother of a teenage son, who is sixteen years old, and a teenage daughter, who is fourteen years old. She has a domestic partner, and the couple has been together for ten years. She has twenty years of experience in her field, works a sixty-hour week, and makes a six-figure annual salary. Her partner is a business executive. Paula's main stressor at home is difficulty showing affection to her partner while convincing her fourteen-year-old, who is fast-becoming wayward, that her mother still loves her despite breaking up with her father. However, that is not her main problem.

Paula's battles with depression started in her early adulthood. Her father neglected her as a child, and her mother raised her in resource-poor conditions. Because of this, she assumed an adult role at a rather early age of sixteen. She ran away from home with a wealthy boyfriend with whom she used and sold illegal drugs and engaged in some other illegal activities that resulted in the loss of lives. She almost emptied one box of tissues as she narrated her ordeal to me. Five years ago, Paula became severely depressed. She denied having nightmares or flashbacks of any past trauma. She became enveloped with a dark cloud of persistent guilt, low self-esteem, hopelessness, pessimism, insomnia, and sadness that never went away. Though she became a Christian and goes to church occasionally, she did not believe that God would ever forgive her because, according to her, her sins were "too grave." Paula denied suicidal ideation.

As I usually do with all my patients, I conducted a thorough psychiatric evaluation with a comprehensive history and made recommendations, but I allowed Paula to determine her preferred treatment approach. She wanted me to leverage all resources available to me in helping her. That is just what I did, and that is what I love to do. I prescribed medications to her. I took her through Christian-based cognitive behavioral therapy. We studied scriptures in the Holy Bible that are key to her healing. We read the scriptures and prayed together on several occasions. After three months of clinical and faith-based interventions, Paula reported to me that her symptoms were completely resolved and that she was more hopeful about her life than she had ever been. Of course, she continues to utilize her treatment plan today with no plans of quitting any time soon.

Just like Paula, there are many people who are merely existing but not thriving. They have thrown in the towel. They have conceded defeat. They are merely spectators in life. Life means nothing to them. They are watching life roll by without the thrill of participating in it. At best, they live their lives in a black and white television mode and never see how colorful life could be. This makes me sad—really sad!

There is Hope!

With that said, I have an obligation to inform you that you have put in far more effort than the average depressed person. The average person with depression is usually unmotivated and is not actively seeking help. The good news is that you are putting in an effort by reading this book. I am glad that you are searching for answers. When I set out to write this book, you are the one I dreamed about. I wanted to write a book that would make a difference in your life. I did a lot of soul-searching. I prayed for direction. I thought of my interactions with the many individuals that I have worked with.

Yes, you are the one I saw. Wherever you are, I want to know that I feel drawn to you. There is a spiritual connection I cannot deny. Initially, I thought that I did not have time in my busy schedule to write a book. Nevertheless, I felt compelled. You may feel like you're sinking into a bottomless pit in quicksand. But wait! Hold on! Help is coming!

Something Must Be Done

Just as I started to write, I heard the news—A seemingly successful healthcare professional, whom I had worked with rather closely, had just taken his own life. I tell myself, "Something must be done!" I feel that time will run out if we do not act swiftly enough.

In the following chapters, I will explore my journey and my unique process for achieving total and lasting healing from depression. I hope that you will find in the following chapters tested, proven, and usable tools that you can apply right away in your life. This book was written with you in mind. It is meant to be a companion to aid you in your journey to total healing and lasting health.

Chapter 2

The Making of a Healer

"The planet does not need more 'successful people.' The planet desperately needs more peacemakers, healers, restorers, storytellers, and lovers of all kinds."
– Dalai Lama

You have heard the saying, "Nothing happens by accident." That is what I had on my mind when I started writing this chapter. Healers are not made in an instant. If you spoke to any healing professional, you would marvel at their respective journeys. It is interesting to note that our journeys are, by themselves, a source of healing. In this chapter, I will share my story with you. You might ask, "Why share your story? Doesn't that make you vulnerable?" Of course, it does, but wait. Will it bring healing? If yes, then isn't it worth sharing? If one man's vulnerability would bring healing to many, then it is a thousand times worth the cost. According to Les Brown, "Telling our stories is an act of generosity."

Coming back to the idea that nothing happens by accident, I am a firm believer in the fact that although our decisions go to shape and color the outcomes we get in life, our lives' journeys are also divinely masterminded. Our lives are a product of this delicate balance. To that effect, I can assure you that if you're reading this book our paths are not crossing by accident. All along, we were meant to be on the journey of life together. All along, my life has been preparing me to become the one who is walking on your emotional journey with you. We should not walk this important journey as strangers. I will share parts of my life's journey with you to help you understand how I came to be with you. I would like you to know the factors that influenced my life's journey and the lessons that I learned along the way. My desire is that you and I can connect on a deeper level.

The Beginning

I was born and raised in Ghana, West Africa. I grew up in a close-knit, lower-middle-income, Christian family that I am truly grateful for. My early childhood years were marked by bittersweet experiences. Being the youngest of my mother's eight children and the seventh of my father's eight children (I hope you can do the math!), I was glad that I had several older siblings, who were successful in their own rights and acted as role models to me, a father who was the headteacher of our primary school and an academic icon in the community, and a mother who is my spiritual tower. However, I had my fair share of emotional difficulties which help me to empathize with those who are hurting. Somewhere along the line, my parents separated for several years, and my older brother and I were raised by our mother who had no profession or financial support.

Let me interrupt that thought and express how much I detest instability in relationships. I cannot finish telling you how many times in my career and ministry that I have heard a story that goes like this, "My childhood was perfect until my parents divorced." I also cannot tell you how many lives have been damaged by relationship break-ups. That is why I am an advocate for healthy relationships. Once a relationship is healthy, it will last, and it will be a source of healing rather than a source of ailment. Healthy relationships are a product of individuals with healthy mindsets, who are fully committed to making things work despite the challenges that they may face. I digress!

For a period of four years, my break-away family unit was enveloped by a cloak of lack and misery. I remember my brother and I waking up each morning and waiting indoors until my mother (who woke up by four o'clock each morning) returned from mending torn clothes for people in our neighborhood for pennies. It was only if she returned home with a few pennies that my brother and I could buy or make breakfast and head off to school. I learned the skill of simultaneously eating breakfast while carrying books on my head and walking to school in the morning. We were only sustained by our solid faith in God that we inherited from our mother. Somehow, even in the midst of these difficulties, I always emerged at the very top of my class in terms of academic performance and personal conduct. Never forget that despite our challenges God always has a special plan for our lives. Never forget that no matter how hopeless your situation becomes God is always up to something!

Later in life, it became clear that God had been preparing me to become an agent of hope and healing to many for years to come. As the years rolled by, I noticed that I repeatedly found myself in situations where I served as a channel of healing and a beacon of hope. It is ironic because I saw myself as the youngest and the least, plus I was an unplanned child, but God had a plan. For the remainder of my years in school, everywhere I went, I naturally assumed the role of a leader. I was selected as class president many times in grade school, senior prefect and students' chaplain in high school, and the president of two student organizations while in college, and I served as a leader at the national level. I found myself delivering vision and a sense of direction to many and I could not escape it.

A Channel of Hope

Many years ago, after completing my first bachelor's degree in Ghana, I worked as an agricultural advisor helping farmers to enhance their livelihoods by growing crops for the export market. I learned a great deal about the process and importance of being an agent of hope. I drove long distances and long hours, often alone, on far-away countryside roads through lush green vegetation. A mission to deliver hope and healing to hurting people fueled me on. For some of my clients, putting one meal on the table (was there even a table?) was a miracle.

Though I am short in stature, the sight of the towering tropical African flora, particularly the Baobab tree, constantly reminded me of my role as a beacon of hope to many. A fully-grown Baobab tree is huge, reaching to about one hundred feet high and thirty-five feet of trunk circumference. I was motivated! I wanted to do more to help my folks. My wife and I, then newly married, went on to England where I obtained my master's degree in agribusiness management at the University of London. After that, the opportunity came for my wife and me to relocate to the United States. At that time, I realized that my mission as a channel of hope and healing had just begun.

Once in the United States, my career took a detour because of an unusual occurrence. While I was in the process of opening my very first U.S. bank account at Chase Bank in Brooklyn, New York, I received an interview on the spot and got a job as a personal banker, moving from first-time bank customer to a banker within hours. Thanks to Dwayne Winter for identifying my potential! That led to my next assignment as a premier client manager and assistant vice president at the Bank of America in West Hartford, Connecticut. I never forgot that I was meant to be a beacon of hope.

In my banking career, I had the privilege of helping individuals and families to plan their finances. This was as exhilarating as it was challenging. You can imagine the culture shock that I experienced moving from helping rural farmers in Africa to helping grow financial wealth in America's financial capital region. Beyond my resilience and my ability to adapt to changing circumstances and beyond my curiosity to learn new concepts and excel, I was determined to put smiles on the faces of my clients. I was virtually a healer in a turbulent financial system as I consistently helped to calm emotions. I enjoyed the adventure and loved my job because I worked directly with individuals to protect and grow something that they treasured—their financial assets. However, I did not find fulfillment in my banking career. I found the banking system to be too aggressive for me, as I was brought up to appreciate humanitarian values over material pursuits.

I did some soul-searching. I wanted to discover the real me so I could become my true self. I remembered that when I was a young boy growing up in Africa, my original dream was to become a medical doctor. I used to joke to my friends, "Medicine or suicide!" Now I know not to make such expensive jokes. After high school, I could not gain admission to medical school. With only two medical schools in Ghana at the time, there was a limited number of openings for a large number of candidates. "What a bummer!" I said to myself. It was at this time that I changed my career plans and studied agriculture for my first degree. While working in banking, I researched ways to accomplish my childhood dream. I did not want to forfeit my income and enroll in medical school. I thought that would be unfair to my young family. I realized that I could become a registered nurse by obtaining another bachelor's degree in nursing, and I could build on that to become a nurse practitioner. As a nurse practitioner, I could take care of patients just like a medical doctor does. Then I would be a true channel of hope and healing. *Viola!* Thank God for America, the land of opportunity!

A New Beginning

It was a Friday afternoon when my new career journey started. I was still working at the Bank of America. I left work early and drove to the University of Connecticut School of Nursing, showed all my previous transcripts to an admissions advisor, and asked how I could get into their accelerated nursing program. I started in my prerequisite classes. Nothing would stop me. As fate would have it, the credit crunch of 2008 hit. The bank laid me off. Instead of being discouraged, I became even more fueled. I had a mission to complete. I thought to myself, "I cannot fail the many hurting people that need what I have to offer." I was finally accepted into nursing school. Anyone who has gone to nursing school in the United States would tell you that it was one of the hardest things that they have ever done.

I have much respect for fellow nurses who survived rigorous academic and clinical storms and are at the forefront of healthcare in America daily! Even more challenging was the accelerated version of nursing school. It was intensive! We had didactics on Fridays from 8:00 a.m. until 6:00 p.m. with a lunch break, and we spent the rest of the week on clinical rotations in various hospitals in Connecticut. During my first clinical training at the Waterbury Hospital in Connecticut, one of my first patients refused to have me (a black nurse) care for her. I will never forget what my instructor advised me to do because it is the very thing I stand for. God bless her. I can still hear her voice. My instructor, Mrs. Carol T. Fray, RN, MSN, APRN, said, "Kill them with love!" Without looking back, I have been killing my patients with love ever since!

Commitment to Christ

One of the aspects of my calling that I have not yet told you is my role in Christian ministry. Serving in church has been an integral part of my life since my teenage years. My father was a Catechist in the Evangelical Presbyterian Church and my mother has always been literally addicted to church and prayer for as far back as I can remember. As a young boy, I carried my mother's heavy Bible on my head as we went to church every morning. At the age of fourteen, I gained a deep, personal understanding of the love of God through Christ and invited Jesus Christ to be my Lord. At that time, I took a personal vow to serve God for the rest of my life. Since then, I have had the privilege of serving in multiple roles in various churches.

One night in the fall of 2010 while speaking to the church, my pastor, Reverend Sampson Yeboah, asked a question that gave birth to what has now become my passion and career. Reverend Sampson asked the church, "Have you noticed that anytime you interact with Brother Joy, you become encouraged?" I was then in nursing school. That night, he opened my eyes to a world of need and opportunity as well as my potential to make a difference. This is what God had been shaping me for all my life. When my family got home that night, my wife asked me, "Haven't you known this all along?" Before I could respond, she added, "Anytime you speak to people, even if they were feeling down, they would be up by the time they're leaving you." There it is! My calling was staring me in the face. I realized that I was a channel of hope and purpose. I thank God for transformational fathers and visionary wives!

Before I graduated from nursing school, I knew that I would spend the rest of my life providing hope, healing, and purpose to others. After I became board-certified as a registered nurse, I worked as a psychiatric and mental health nurse for several years in two regional teaching hospitals in Connecticut while pursuing my second graduate studies in psychiatric nursing. I served passionately at the bedside of those who were hopeless. I listened to the grieving with empathy. I administered medications to the hurting. I was a light brightening the path of the confused and bringing clarity of thought to the frustrated. I served as a charge nurse and nurse preceptor, bringing the best out of budding healers.

It has always been my personal philosophy that "if it must be done, then it must be done well." Fueled by this conviction, I enrolled in the University of South Alabama College of Nursing Master of Science and Doctor of Nursing Practice dual degree program that took me four gruesome years to complete. Just like other would-be nurse practitioners, I was expected to become as clinically knowledgeable as I was kind and caring. The program emphasized critical thinking and appropriate judgment while working with the individuals that we served. For my clinical practicum, I worked with several seasoned preceptors at reputable hospitals and outpatient clinics including the Community Mental Health Affiliates (CMHA) in New Britain, Connecticut, The Hospital at Hebrew Senior Care in Bloomfield, Connecticut, and Newington Internal Medicine, in Newington, Connecticut. My preceptors included experienced psychiatrist nurse practitioners and psychiatrists. I sat for and passed the national board certification exam via the American Nurses Credentialing Center (ANCC) to become a psychiatric and mental health nurse practitioner (PMHNP-BC). This part of my journey ended with a doctoral residency at the Cope Community Services, Inc. in Tucson, Arizona.

When I started my career as a nurse practitioner, I first worked in the corrections field where I mainly prescribed medications for inmates at a county jail. After that, I cared for individuals at a community mental health outpatient clinic where I practiced alongside several other psychiatric providers. A few nights a week, I provide emergency psychiatric stabilization services at the Crisis Response Center in Tucson where I work with individuals who are in danger of harming themselves or others either due to suicidal or homicidal ideation, psychosis, or substance abuse. I also serve as a member of the Medical Executive Committee where I contribute in the areas of developing clinical policies and reviewing my peers.

My Pastoral Ministry

Somewhere along the line, I completed a pastoral training and became ordained as Christian minister in the state of Arizona. With the help of my wife and a few friends, I started a vibrant Christian Charismatic church in Tucson, Arizona, the Impact Chapel of the International Central Gospel Church (ICGC), where I volunteer my services as the senior pastor. My pastoral duties include preparing and delivering sermons, teaching, counseling, and discipling others. As a Christian minister, my passion is to ensure that as many people as possible will find their place in the kingdom of God and fulfill their destinies on earth. I want as many people as possible to hear the following words of approval from God at the end of their lives:

"… Well done, good and faithful servant; you have been faithful over a few things. I will make you ruler over many things. Enter into the joy of your lord" (Matthew 25:23).

My sermons can be summed up into a ten-fold message, namely repentance from sin and eternal life by salvation through Christ; personal life-long relationship with God and dominion over the flesh; generosity in giving and in serving others in and outside the church; accepting and maintaining healthy relationships with all people; strengthening the weak and freeing the oppressed; healing and health for the body and liberty for the mind; hope for the future and abundant life in Christ; prosperity through honest labor and blessings of God; success by discovering, developing, and deploying one's calling; and positioning the church as a family of Christians and a training ground where we learn to believe in God, belong to a caring family, become all that God wants us to be, and build the kingdom of God on earth.

These rich experiences naturally led me to start a private mental health practice called the Tucson Treatment Center, Inc. (TTC) in 2017. Seeing people at my private practice permits me to fully express myself and my beliefs in a unique way. In the spirit of client-centered care, I am able to veer off traditional treatment trajectories and venture into areas that each individual is interested in without excessive organizational restrictions. In other words, I can use as many tools or as few tools as my clients are willing to use. For the past two years at TTC, I have worked with individuals who are struggling with mood disorders such as depression, anxiety, bipolar disorder, post-traumatic stress disorder, obsessive-compulsive disorder, and psychotic disorders.

I know I am making a difference in the lives of people when someone enters my office for a follow-up appointment and exclaims, "Oh my gosh, Dr. Joy, you changed my life!"

This always brings tears to my eyes. I often feel bittersweet when a patient leaves my office and says, "Thank you, Dr. Joy. You're the first doctor that has taken the time to listen to me." I wonder where our healthcare system is headed as doctors are increasingly unable to spend quality time with their patients. Having grown up in Africa, my natural disposition is based on the time-tested values of caring for others. This is a concept called "Ubuntu," a Southern African term meaning, "I am because we are." It is this universal bond of sharing that informs my philosophy of practice.

The Next Chapter

Within the past few years, I have had an awakening as I either worked with or heard about many leaders in business, in healthcare, in academia, and even in the church, who have either taken their own lives or are struggling under the weight of depression and anxiety. I am hoping that by the grace of God, I can devote the next phase of my career to working with this important population while also speaking to audiences in a quest to find total and permanent healing for mood disorders. So, you see? For all of my life, I have been preparing for this moment— to bring hope and healing to you. I hope that this book will be a tool that will deliver healing, hope, joy, and fulfillment into your life. Let's dive into the meat of my healing process.

Chapter 3

The Authentic Healing Process

"Ultimate cure is only possible when we treat the person as a whole, not just the 'hole' in the person."

How does depression come about? Depression may be caused by several factors. Depression may be caused by biological factors such as hereditary or genetic factors where it runs in one's family, unexplained neurological factors where chemical imbalances or other abnormalities develop in the brain; or situational factors where adverse life experiences, such as failure, losses, disappointment, or lack of fulfillment in life may be responsible. Depression may be caused by any combination of these and/or other causes that were not mentioned here. As evident in some sacred books, demonic activity is another possible cause of disease.[4] Although it is not always possible to determine what caused an individual's depression, psychiatric providers regularly conduct a thorough evaluation to narrow down the root cause(s) as much as possible so we can develop a treatment plan that is individualized and responsive.

To that effect, majority of the psychiatry and psychology community agrees that the best way to approach depression is to adopt a multi-faceted approach that leverages several interventions in a holistic fashion. However, only a few interventions (pharmacotherapy and psychotherapy) are routinely used in most psychiatric clinics and doctors' offices around the world. The question is, "Why are we leaving some interventions unused?" Many reasons may exist for this great omission. I believe one of the main reasons why some potentially effective tools (such as exercise, nutrition, and prayer) are not used in a typical psychiatry office is that our healthcare systems are fashioned to promote only a few interventions. In the United States, for example, most commercial health insurance plans may not pay for a professional, who sees patients for the purpose of prayer as an intervention for depression. The very training of psychiatric providers does not cover the development of expertise in spiritual interventions, exercise interventions, or nutritional remedies for depression. These aspects are left for other experts who specialize in those areas. We forget that those experts are often not in our psychiatry offices and are not typically involved in care planning for our patients, neither do we go out of our way to bring them in. Maybe it is too much work? It was in response to this that I developed my treatment process.

The Authentic Healing Process for Depression (AHPD)

In this chapter, I will give you an overview of the Authentic Healing Process for Depression (AHPD). This is a process that I had to develop as a response to the fragmentation mentioned above. It came about rather organically. I utilize parts of the AHPD in my practice and this has helped me and my partners to test its effectiveness in a crude form and fine-tune it into an efficacious system of healing from depression. I developed the AHPD because, although a good number of people recover from depression through the existing traditional approaches, psychiatric providers continue to see in clinical practice a large number of people who do not respond to conventional psychiatry. By traditional approaches or conventional psychiatry, I mean the use of medications and/or psychotherapy only. In the United States, these two interventions are the most commonly used in the treatment of depression. From time to time, providers employ additional interventions mostly in the form of recommendations for exercising regularly and getting adequate sleep and maintaining a healthy diet. These additional interventions are typically not incorporated into treatment plans in a coherent fashion. Providers usually leave these interventions as mere recommendations for the patient to consider.

Let's consider the best results that we obtain from our current treatment approaches. A patient goes to see a psychiatric provider, obtains an evaluation and treatment recommendations, and initiates treatment. After a period of say six months to a year of treatment, this individual returns to the provider and states, "Hi Doc! I am cured! I am not depressed anymore!" A discussion is then held regarding whether the individual needs to remain on medication or not. Believe it or not, we get such results often. Most outcomes fall somewhere on a spectrum with a majority of our patients coming back to say, "Hello Doctor, I am feeling somewhat better, but my depression has not gone away." Research has shown that less than fifty per cent of individuals respond to first line antidepressant treatment or psychotherapy.[5]

Even if the individual is fortunate enough to obtain the best results described above, this result is still a clinical success only. This book is about total healing, meaning healing of the entire person inside out—spirit, soul, and body. Whenever one of my patients comes back to me with great clinical outcomes, of course, we do a happy dance together and celebrate. After this celebration, I often ask myself, "Is that all?" What if the symptoms return in six months? What can this person do to maintain the gains that were made?

Even in the best-case scenario, let's assume that the individual lives for the rest of his or her life free from depression—awesome! Many from the clinical community would consider this the best thing that can ever happen to a depressed patient. But, is that all life is about? What is this person's destiny? What about her soul? Should we only heal the body and send our patients on their way or should we care about the whole person? It is at this point that my spiritual insight kicks in. These are the questions and factors that provoked me to develop the AHPD. If I am going to be an effective healing professional, I must care about the entire person.

The foundational principle of the AHPD is the fact that man is a spirit that lives in a body and has a soul. This means that we are not the physical body that is visible. Your body is the container/housing that you live in. Your soul is an immaterial part of you that helps you to function here on earth. At the basic level, we can say that we are made of three integrated components: spirit, soul, and body. Because of this integration, any time one component of man becomes injured, the other components are affected as well. With this understanding, it is obvious that if a treatment approach to depression is going to be effective, it must address all three components of man in a coherent fashion.

On that basis, I went on a mission to formulate a framework for treating and healing depression truthfully and in an authentic manner. I wanted a process that would get the job done for good. I wanted a one-stop shop for healing depression. I know that this will take many lifetimes to fully accomplish, but I have a workable framework at this time that gets results and must be shared.

Theoretical Basis

The theoretical underpinning for the AHPD is the biopsychosocial model of healthcare which was developed by George L. Engel,[6] a spiritual dimension from my ministry experience, and self-efficacy dimension based on work done by Albert Bandura.[7] The blended theoretical basis is the biopsychosocial-spiritual model. The AHPD is based on the understanding that human beings are not only biological and psychological, but we are also social and spiritual. This process helps psychiatric healing professionals to view our patients as whole entities and not physical beings only. This is the missing link that exists in the traditional biomedical treatment of depression.

For me, it was like a light switch that turned on. My desire for authentic healing from depression led me to research and develop the AHPD into its current form. I have repeatedly used the AHPD with some of my patients and the results have been phenomenal. I have included the current framework below (See Figure 1).

Figure 1: The Authentic Healing Process for Depression (AHPD)

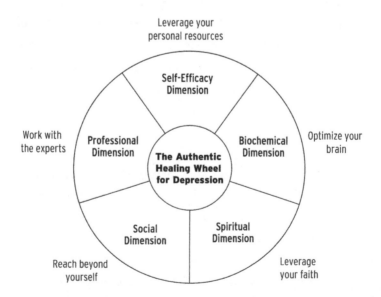

I have named this treatment approach the Authentic Healing Process for Depression (AHPD) for many reasons. I wanted to develop a process that gets lasting results. I wanted to make sure that the process that I came up with was true to the core. I wanted my process to be genuine and effective, even if it requires tremendous effort. I wanted to make sure that the results obtained through this process were authentic. There are times when we buy an item from the store, take it home, start using it, and realize that it does get results, but those results are short-lived. They soon fade away, and the item becomes obsolete. Such an item is not authentic. In the same way, there are times when people begin to feel better after starting treatment for depression. Some people may even overcome depression for good only to realize that our true victory does not lie in our ability to overcome depression alone. There is more to life than becoming depression-free. The AHPD addresses your entire journey from where you are to a place where you will be truly fulfilled in life. I cannot emphasize this enough.

If there is anything you should take away from this book, this is it: True victory over depression—or any ailment for that matter—lies in our ability to have total healing and lifelong fulfillment, with or without the symptoms that we may have been dealing with in the first place. I know you're asking yourself, "What do you mean?" This is what I mean: Yes, you can heal from depression, and I will help with that, but is that what matters most in life? Next time it might be fibromyalgia. Then it might be cancer. I pray that that will not be your story, but the point is that each person is facing multiple challenges in life, making it imperative for us to move away from fragmented methods of healing and to more holistic or integrative approaches. By total healing, I mean healing of your spirit, soul, and body.

Life is said to be a problem-solving process. So long as we are alive, we will encounter problems every day. Our ability to thrive lies not in solving one problem but in mastering the skill of solving any problem that comes our way and remaining victorious ever after. In other words, I ask you to lift up your game! Of course, this book will show you how to overcome depression, but that is not all there is in life. What is the point in escaping from a sinking ship only to get killed by fire in a rescue boat? I want to work with people who are depressed today and guide them to become truly fulfilled and victorious. To me, that is what it means to be a channel of hope and purpose.

The Five Domains

As you can see in Figure 1, the AHPD is made up of five domains (or areas of focus)—the area of self-efficacy, the biochemical area, the spiritual area, the social area, and the professional area. In this context, self-efficacy is one's belief in one's potential to heal and one's ability to harness that conviction in the healing process. Every one of us is equipped with enough substance to power our own healing. Self-efficacy is the backbone for your healing, the engine room in which your healing takes place. The stronger your self-efficacy, the more likely you are to heal. In other words, a person who does not believe that he or she will heal is not likely to heal. In the next chapter of this book, we will cover the area of self-efficacy more exhaustively.

The next component of the AHPD is the biochemical area. Research has shown that there are differences in chemical composition in the brains of individuals who are clinically depressed when compared with individuals who are not.[8] One of the well-known differences is that people who are depressed appear to have lower levels of the neurotransmitters serotonin, norepinephrine, and dopamine than people who are not depressed.[9] In the biochemical area of the AHPD, the goal is to leverage the many resources that are known to increase the levels of these neurotransmitters in the brain, promote the growth of brain cells, and enhance communication among brain cells in the individual who is depressed.

The third component of the AHPD is the spiritual area. Although human beings have tremendous internal resources that can be leveraged for healing, we are limited in how much we can do. Our universe provides us with multitudes of proofs that there is a higher power through whom our world came to be and who sustains us. We call this higher power God. He made us and He sure has the power to fix us when we are broken. Friend, our focus in the spiritual area is to leverage the healing power of God, enjoy the unadulterated love that He demonstrates to us, and tap into His immeasurable ability to transform our destinies.

Next, the social area of the AHPD is obviously the area that helps us to level healing from the interconnections that we have with other humans. Believe it or not, there is as much healing in relationships as there are in medications. However, this source of healing must be nurtured and leveraged.

The last domain of the AHPD is the professional area. In this domain, we will explore all the benefits that working with mental health professionals can bring to you as you embark on your journey to overcome depression. In the next several chapters, we will discuss each of the AHPD areas in more detail, starting with the area of self-efficacy.

The Retired Healthcare Professional

It will interest you to know that healers and solution-givers also need healing some of the time. When this happens, open-mindedness and creativity are required on the part of the care provider. Bennet is a male, Caucasian retired psychiatric nurse practitioner whom I have been treating for depression for a few years now. He asked me to include his story in my book so others can learn from his experience with finding a cure for depression.

"At age sixty-one, I am grateful for my own unique path. It has been unpredictable, novel, and every day I cherish life despite my psychiatric and other health challenges. My work as a nurse and nurse practitioner served me well. I learned that I had strengths unknown to me. Every patient I encountered taught me more about myself and challenged me physically, mentally, and spiritually. These experiences formed who I am and made me a better, kinder person."

"While I have two master's degrees and am well-educated, one particular patient taught me many things that I did not know from academia. She had anxiety and depression and battled daily with depersonalization secondary to a history of sexual abuse. My usual approaches and short-term solutions didn't work. She wore dark glasses for all sessions. We had hour-long sessions, and we walked in a park as she felt, being overweight, uncomfortable sitting across the table from me. It took a while, but with critical thinking, thinking outside of the box, and creativity, I helped her to overcome her mood problems. Later on, when my own depression became worse and I came to see Dr. Joy, I saw the same exact qualities in him. It appeared as if we went through the same school of life. He showed and continues to demonstrate genuine flexibility, understanding, creativity, empathy, and the willingness to integrate varying and unconventional approaches to managing my symptoms. No wonder I am in a stable place today."

Chapter 4

The Self-Efficacy Dimension

*"Whether you think you can, or
you think you can't, you're right."*
– Henry Ford

The self-efficacy dimension of the Authentic Healing Process for Depression (AHPD) is based on the concept that healing starts with the divinely empowered self. It is your perception of your ability to heal. It is your level of confidence in your ability to heal. Just like any other major undertaking, healing begins from the known (where you are right now) to the unknown (where you want to be—healed!). You have heard that charity begins at home. Similarly, your healing begins with you, not as a self-sufficient entity but as an entity that can leverage internal and external resources to achieve lasting healing. Albert Bandura is the developer of the original concept of self-efficacy. He is a Canadian-American scholar who is considered to be the greatest living psychologist of our times.[10] According to Bandura, "Persons who have a strong sense of efficacy deploy their attention and effort to the demands of the situation and are spurred by obstacles to greater effort."[11] In the context of this book, self-efficacy is not independent of God. I must be emphasized that without God, you can accomplish nothing.

The Deception of Depression

Believe it or not, when empowered by God, you are capable of more than you think. In my life, I have noticed that the average person tends to think or believe less about themselves than they should—Thanks to the societal virtue of modesty. As if this is not bad enough, depression comes to make this lack of self-confidence a thousand times worse. Low self-esteem is one of the cardinal symptoms of depression. When people get depressed, their estimation of themselves virtually plunges into the lowest levels. Depression makes you believe that everyone else is happy except you. Depression makes you believe the worst things about yourself—and guess what, most of it is untrue. The language of depression is, "I am the only one in this situation. I am the odd one out. I am a terrible person. There is no hope for me."

What you need to know is that the voice of depression is different from your voice. You and depression are separate entities. Don't make the mistake of owning depression. Depression is an unwelcome guest that seeks to dominate your life. If you carefully listen to yourself speak, you will admit that you are not the one speaking. It is the depression inside of you that is speaking. I often hear people speak like, "I am bipolar." I would like to believe that this is only a figure of speech and not an act of owning the illness. Your ability to separate yourself from your illnesses is fundamental to your ability to heal.

Simply put, the human being is a divine masterpiece! If a human being were to be placed in a ranking with the most powerful inventions in history, man would break the chart, as we are in our own category. This is what the writer of the Book of Psalms realized when he wrote Psalm 139:14:

"I will praise You, for I am fearfully and wonderfully made; Marvelous are Your works…"

You were supernaturally and intricately engineered with parts that are far more phenomenal than meets the eye. Your very make-up is incomprehensible. In God, your potential and abilities are unfathomable. Your potential to tap into your Maker's ability to heal and recover, your divine ability to bounce back and soar high, and your God-given ability to defy and redefine the norm is out of this world! Scientists have barely scratched the surface in discovering the divinely endowed potential of the human. That is who you are!

Becoming self-efficacious does not mean that you should go through life with a false sense of self-esteem, claiming that everything is alright while there are major problems staring you in the face or bubbling beneath. This is true for some of the high-achieving individuals that I have worked with. They forget that even masterpieces suffer damage from time to time. You don't want to continue to pretend as if everything is alright when it is not. I know you often put up a show for others only to crash when you're by yourself. However, it is one thing lying to others and an entirely different thing lying to yourself. You are the last person you want to ever lie to. If you are depressed or emotionally impaired in some way, the very first thing you must do is to admit to yourself that something is wrong and must be addressed. This is because you can never solve a problem that you do not acknowledge in the first place. Yes, acknowledge it but don't own it.

Self-Efficacy in Action

Janelle is one of my business partners. She is in her early twenties. She was in the military when she slipped into a depressive episode after a significant traumatic event. She began isolating from her friends and lost her drive for completing everyday tasks. Her work ethic diminished. This affected her mood and behavior at work. She was agitated easily and then would be tearful due to feeling guilty for her behaviors. She experienced feelings of failure, emptiness, and low self-esteem. She lacked in the area of spirituality, however, she had social connections that were continuously checking in on her whenever she tried to isolate.

Janelle's saving grace was the strong self-efficacy that she instilled. Somehow, she was able to identify the reason why she was feeling angry or irritable. She then confided in friends. She changed how she spoke to herself in her mind when she felt like she was failing. Instead of stating, "This depression will never end," she began to tell herself, "There are ways to feel okay even when I am failing." This individual focused on her strengths and she used positive and truthful statements about herself and her situation to generate the energy and peace that she needed to keep moving on. She kept working on herself while depending on God. Her insight saved her from the dangers of pessimism and the tendency to blame others for her predicament. She knew that she needed to do a lot of work on herself in order to sustain the progress she was making. The result was decreased anger, enhanced positive self-image and improved interactions with coworkers, and a better mood overall. This is what self-efficacy can do.[12]

The Plight of Leaders

Coming back to my fellow leaders—because of your track record of successes, others might have come to know you as a strong person, so you tend to live with the false idea that you must remain strong, even when you are weak. You convince yourself that you would let your followers down if you admit that you are weak and need help. You must "dress up" for the cameras. This may be one of the reasons for the rising rate of suicide among celebrities and leaders.

If you are one of such people, you probably drink alcohol or use other intoxicating substances to help you to forget about it all or become numb to the problem. Doing so will only put a tape on the problem for a short period of time, and the problem will resurface later, often in a more complex form than before. Archbishop Duncan Williams once stated, "The serpent that Adam and Eve failed to kill in the Book of Genesis later became the dragon in the Book of Revelation." I hope and pray that you will not fall prey to this unhealthy delay.

Acknowledging that you are depressed and need help is an internal work in which you defy your ego and initiate the process of healing. You're literally saying, "Ouch! This hurts! And it is embarrassing, but I must talk to someone about it!" Admitting that there is a problem does not make you a weak person. In fact, our society got it all wrong—People who are afflicted with depression are not weak people. We must talk about depression until it becomes a household subject. We must talk about it until it loses its cloak of invincibility. Can you imagine if someone was drowning in body of water but failed to scream or disturb the water because he did not want to be noticed? That person would surely drown. Acknowledging that there is an impairment gives you the opportunity to begin your healing journey. Welcome to the club of broken masterpieces called humans!

The Cost of Depression

Next, if you are going to achieve lasting healing, you need to estimate how much it is costing you to remain depressed. Have you ever thought about that? This is important because, if your situation feels normal to you, you may not have the urgency or motivation that is needed to fix it. When you count the cost, you would realize that depression is quite an expensive undertaking.

The economic burden of depression is revealed in the fact that the United States alone loses about $210.5 billion to depression each year.[13] The cost of depression can be seen in the number of days you take off from work, the fact that you're less productive, the lost precious family and fun times, the joy you miss in relationships because you tend to isolate from others, etc. Some people have lost a potential spouse or business partner only because they have a cloak of depression covering their true charm. As beautiful as you are, depression has a way of inhibiting you in such a way that you neglect self-care which is meant to reveal your beauty and you avoid social connections where your beauty finds its expression. Depression also robs you of your ability to express your intelligence. Could this be the reason you lost that contract or job opportunity?

Analyze Your Strengths and Weaknesses

Analyzing your strengths and weaknesses is an important activity in your journey to becoming self-efficacious. Yes, everyone has strengths, and everyone has weaknesses. These are going to be important in your healing journey. You may be asking yourself, "Me? Strengths?" The reason you ask is that depression has damaged your self-confidence to the point where you are blind to your strengths and you have stopped believing in yourself. Your strengths are reflected in things that you do in your life without much effort. Your weaknesses are areas in which you struggle without many results, even with maximum effort. Your strengths and weaknesses are what make you unique. Your difference or uniqueness is a key to your success in life.

In the fall of 2017, a woman walked into my office for an initial psychiatric diagnostic evaluation. I will call her Emily. She looked shy. Though fifty-one, Emily acted as a twenty-five-year-old. She was dealing with depression and anxiety. Her leading symptoms were low self-esteem, excessive guilt, isolation, lack of motivation, poor concentration, restlessness, and tremors. You would expect that a professor and researcher at a leading university would be more confident, but she had zero self-confidence.

As we talked, it became obvious that Emily was a middle child with an older brother and a younger sister. Her siblings have always been over-achievers. Emily is not. She reported that her parents always compared her with her siblings, constantly reminding her that even her younger sister was doing better in school and in life. Emily is unique. She reported to me that she takes things at her own pace. She said, "I get done when I get done." Soon after she was offered a job at the university, her fiancé broke up with her, bringing back her childhood memories that she was not good enough. She was out of work for three days prior to coming to see me as "I just couldn't pick myself up," per Emily. I realized that she needed to do some work in the area of self-efficacy.

After an elaborate assessment, we developed and launched a treatment plan that included Christian cognitive behavioral therapy, fifteen milligrams of Buspirone twice daily, and self-confidence building exercises. After eight weeks of implementing this plan, Emily started to bounce back. Her affect became brighter and her self-confidence soared. After three months, her work productivity soared, and she was ready to date again. She became more motivated to pursue her life's mission of raising researchers that are at the cutting edge of their areas of specialization.

Similarly, identifying, pursuing, and fulfilling your calling is a master key to healing from depression and living a truly joy-filled life. Everyone, including you, has a calling or a life mission depending on how you choose to call it. Your calling is your purpose on earth. Your calling is the assignment that you need to complete in order to be truly fulfilled in your life and gain the approval of your maker. In my short life, I noticed that people who have a clear sense of purpose tend to be highly energized. On the other hand, people who do not know their calling are often sad, empty, unmotivated, and lethargic. If you are going to truly heal from depression, you must dare to discover, develop, and deploy your mission in life. I teach quite extensively on this subject from my pulpit at the ICGC Impact Chapel in Tucson, Arizona.

To discover your calling, you must first ask your Creator. He made you. He must know why He made you. He will either tell you or show you your calling, or He will guide you into your calling. Secondly, you may undergo a personal assessment where you ask yourself and answer several soul-searching questions, such as, "What am I passionate about? What causes me to lose sleep? What am I naturally good at? What do I excel in? What do I often lose track of time doing? What lights me up? When a discussion is going on around me, what subject catches my attention more than the others?" Answers to these questions will help you narrow down and discover your purpose. Additionally, ask the people around you for feedback, as they often know you more than you think.

Another interesting way to discover your calling is to get busy doing whatever is presented to you and trust God to lead you along His chosen path for your life. Our God is a skillful shepherd, who is known for picking up people from where they are to where they need to be. He has a track record in this area, and you can believe Him to do that with you. Both in Biblical times and in our times, many people found their calling by serving under another person who is busy delivering on his or her calling. While doing this, before long, your calling will emerge. Referring to how important your purpose is in difficult times, Dr. Myles Munroe said, "Joy in the midst of hell is the hallmark of those who have truly found God's purpose for their lives." Finding your purpose can have an effect on your mood comparable to taking Prozac.

After you discover your calling, please go the extra mile and write it down. There is a supernatural power built into every vision that is written down and plainly expressed. O my! I cannot emphasize this enough! You must do it to experience the power in it. Habakkuk 2:2 says, "Write the vision, and make it plain on tablets that he may run who reads it." Don't miss out on this! I can't wait to hear about the successes that you are achieving as you do this. Finally, break down your overall mission into smaller achievable goals, put a timeline to their accomplishment, and initiate your pursuit from the point closest to you. You may not be able to execute according to the timelines you set, but I have noticed that written down goals placed on a schedule have a far higher chance of inspiring action than those that have not been placed on a schedule.

At the age of twenty-five, I was a young college graduate who was barely starting out in life. One day, as I walked down the street, I saw a beautiful picture that was being offered for sale by a street vendor in Accra, the capital city of Ghana. It looked like the kind of future that I would like to have for myself and my family. It was an attractive depiction of a mansion built on a hill with a red sports car parked in the driveway, enveloped by carefully manicured green lawns, and healthy children playing in the yard. Instantly, I felt connected to it. As you can imagine, I bought it and hung it on my bedroom wall right next to my fiancée's picture, which was already up. I noticed that anytime I woke up in the morning, I was full of energy, and I was quick to jump out of bed. Later, I realized that there was an inherent energizing power in my wall hangings that literally kicked me out of bed each morning for several years. No wonder I did not have any problem getting motivated. Several years later, I can say to the glory of God that my life began to look pretty close to what I had been feeding my eyes on. Friend, what are you feeding your eyes and mind on? I challenge you: Dare to feast your eyes on the future you desire for yourself and see miracles happen in your life!

The Power of the Mind

Psychology is an interplay of how the human mind affects human behavior. It can be infuriating when a depressed person is told, "It's all in your mind." However, a lot of what you experience in your mood and your behaviors can be traced back to the way your mind works. Isn't that why this area of study is called mental health? The television preacher Joyce Meyer says that the human mind is a battlefield. Battles are not fought leisurely. That means you must approach this area with all seriousness. For authentic emotional healing to take place, the mind must first be healed.

Your mind is the womb of your emotions. The Holy Bible states in Proverbs 23:7a, *"For as he thinks in his heart, so is he…"* The Holy Book also says in Proverbs 4:23, *"Keep your heart with all diligence, for out of it spring the issues of life."* By *heart*, the scripture is referring to your innermost part or your core. Finally, the scripture instructs us in Romans 12:2 to "… *be transformed by the renewing of your mind…*" You see, renewing your mind will initiate or expedite your healing. The issues of life, including depression and anxiety, as well as healing from them, all originate from the core of your being. Safeguard this area with all your strength.

How do you renew your mind? By feeding it repeatedly with the right material! You can call it detoxing and reprogramming your mind if you like. It is important that you deliberately select what material goes into your mind and what does not. I realized that several people are depressed because of the series of bad news they are bombarded with day in, day out. Unfortunately, many people are wholesale consumers of information rather than selective consumers. Many patients who come into my office in a worse mood than usual confess to me that they had been watching the news, and they would often add, "The news is quite depressing." That is where positive affirmations come into play. Hang tight. I will address the aspect of affirmations in more detail in the chapter on spirituality. In all your efforts, remember to leverage your personal resources while depending on your Source.

Chapter 5

The Biochemical
Dimension

*"Any man could, if he were so inclined,
be the sculptor of his own brain."*
— Santiago Ramon y Cajal

The biochemical dimension of the AHPD has to do with optimizing your brain. Our focus here is to identify what you need to do to improve the health of your brain in order to heal from depression. Depression is a rather complex illness. Depression may occur because your brain is not producing as many neurons (cells) as it should. Depression may occur because the neurons in your brain are not communicating with one another as much as they should. However, one of the most common factors that has been linked to depression is chemical imbalances in your brain.

You probably know that there are chemicals in your brain that influence the way you feel (your mood) and the way you behave. These chemicals are actually chemical messengers called neurotransmitters. Anytime these chemical messengers get out of balance or are unable to move around as freely as originally designed, it is as if a switch has been turned off, and your mood and/or behaviors will change accordingly. It is therefore important to keep re-balancing these chemicals from time to time. Though your brain is naturally wired to re-balance its own processes, many factors can diminish its ability to do so, including genetic factors, medical conditions, trauma, stress, or medications.

Neurotransmitters

The following are the major neurotransmitters that are known to play a role in regulating depressed mood:

1. Serotonin: Serotonin is a chemical messenger that works to regulate mood, appetite, sleep, and pain. Inadequate amounts of serotonin in the brain have been linked to depressed mood, anxiety, panic, insomnia, pain, low appetite, anger, and other mood problems. Because of this, serotonin is one of the main neurotransmitters that we seek to balance out in the healing of depression.

2. Norepinephrine: Norepinephrine has an activating effect on mood and is believed to play a role in regulating motivation, memory, and reward.

3. Dopamine: This neurotransmitter plays a role in movement, motivation, reward, and perception of reality.

4. Acetylcholine: This neurotransmitter plays roles in improving memory and learning.

5. Glutamate: This is the main excitatory neurotransmitter in the brain. It is known to play roles in both depression and bipolar disorder, and it is the target for ketamine, which has been recently approved by the FDA for the treatment of treatment-resistant major depressive disorder (MDD).

6. Gamma-aminobutyric acid (GABA): GABA is the main inhibitory neurotransmitter in the brain. It plays a leading role in keeping you calm. Low levels of GABA are linked to both depression and anxiety.

Several other neurotransmitters and hormones may be involved in bringing about or relieving depression to varying degrees. For instance, a high level of the stress hormone cortisol, which flights against inflammatory processes in the body, has also been linked to depression.[14]

The focus of the biochemical dimension of AHPD is to manipulate the biological and chemical processes in your brain in order to produce rapid and sustained healing. Any activity that stimulates the production of brain cells (neurogenesis) and enhances the balance of neurotransmitters in your brain will also optimize your brain function and expedite your healing from depression. These include abstaining from substances of abuse, maintaining a healthy diet, engaging in regular physical exercise, getting adequate sleep and rest, taking antidepressants as prescribed, and using complementary, alternative, or other interventions.

Abstaining from Substances of Abuse

The first intervention that you need to observe is to seek help to eliminate any substances of abuse in your life if that is a problem area for you. Starting from excessive caffeine drinking, tobacco use, and alcohol abuse to abusing prescribed or illegal drugs. These unhealthy habits produce adverse biochemical changes in the brain and have negative psychological effects on the body that worsen depression. If necessary, you may need to take some time off to get help at a substance abuse rehab.

Maintaining a Healthy Diet

Nutrition has been closely linked with mood in many ways. Too much or too little sugar intake, too high and too low intake of processed carbohydrates or fatty foods, as well as starving, and eating large meals have all been linked to poor mood outcomes. For instance, excessive intake of processed and simple sugars such as sodas may produce a rapid rise in blood glucose. This stimulates the release of insulin into the blood to metabolize the glucose, resulting in a crash and low mood soon thereafter. This produces or worsens mood swings. As much as possible, avoid sugar-containing liquids. Diets that are rich in green leafy vegetables, whole proteins, and complex carbohydrates are preferred. A general guideline is to have three medium-sized meals a day with about two healthy snacks and a lot of water.

My primary care doctor, Dr. Cohen, tells me, "Eat fish, chicken, eggs, nuts, green vegetables, fresh fruits—not dried fruits and not fruit juices." Avoid bread (especially white bread), pasta, cereals, corn, potatoes, fries, tortillas, chips, rice (especially white rice) sodas, candy, and beer. The DASH (Dietary

Approaches to Stop Hypertension) diet and the Mediterranean diet have been shown to be particularly helpful in protecting against depression. Both diets are rich in fruits, vegetables, nuts, beans, seeds, and healthy fats as well as whole grains, fish, with limited amounts of poultry, red meat, and dairy.[15]

A National Institutes of Aging-funded study conducted at the Rush University Medical Center in 2018 evaluated a total of nine hundred and sixty-four participants with an average age of eighty-one annually for approximately six-and-a-half years. Each participant was monitored for symptoms of depression and filled out questionnaires about how often they ate various foods. This study concluded that individuals, who followed a DASH-style diet were eleven percent less likely to develop depression than participants in the group that followed the Western-style diet that is high in saturated fats and sugar.[16]

Water Consumption

Both adequate and regular consumption of water will make significant improvements in your mood. This is because sixty percent of your body, over seventy percent of your brain, and over eighty percent of your lungs are made up of water. Your body needs water to distribute Oxygen and the much-needed nutrients to your brain. Your body also needs water to eliminate toxic wastes from your system. The more you drink, the thinner your blood and the easier it would be for your heart to function.

For optimal physical and mental health, aim at drinking about half your body weight of water in ounces. For instance, if you weigh two hundred pounds, you should aim at drinking about one hundred ounces of water daily. You're going to like this—If you drink alcohol or coffee, you will need to consume even more water than the average person as these fluids make you urinate more.

Physical Exercise

Regular exercise is a game-changer when it comes to healing from depression and living a depression-free life. Several large research studies have shown that regular aerobic exercise produces about the same healing effect as antidepressants and anti-anxiety medications among people who have mild to moderate depression.[17] It is said that the more you move, the better your mood. At the very basic level, this is because physical exercise enhances your blood-flow significantly, and this ensures that the much-needed oxygen and nutrients get to your brain promptly and in the right amounts and toxic substances are promptly expelled from your body as well. Exercise has been shown to play a major role in enhancing neurogenesis and increasing serotonin levels.[18] When this happens regularly, your brain becomes happier, you can think more clearly, and you interpret stressors more appropriately without getting overwhelmed.

I know you're asking, "What kind of exercise and how much exercise are we talking about here?" You first need to check in with your primary care doctor about what you can safely tolerate without compromising your health. However, exercise that involves moderate exertion for twenty to thirty minutes daily for three to four times per week may be appropriate for the average adult who is in good health. Moderate exertion means that while engaged in this exercise, you can talk but it is hard to maintain a conversation as you're panting. My favorite is dancing to loud music. Walking the dog may not be enough. Sorry!

Whenever possible, plan to exercise outdoors during the day as frequently as possible because exposure to bright light and vitamin D have both been noted to enhance mood. With the continuing increase in technology, more and more people are becoming less and less exposed to sunlight, which could be a factor in the increasing rates of depression in most societies today. The following case illustrates the importance of exercise and nutrition in the treatment of depression.

Bernice is a fifty-three-year-old female lawyer who came to see one of my partners. Her experience with depression started in her mid-teens and for the last four years had been constant. She had been treated with Fluoxetine, Venlafaxine, and Mirtazapine at different times, which she reported brought her marginal but sustained benefits. Her medications, however, caused her to gain weight, making her depressive symptoms worse. My partner decided to add an adjunctive therapy of physical activity and nutrition to her treatment plan. What a life saver! Her new treatment included an exercise plan of cardiovascular workouts with moderate weight and strength training lasting thirty to forty-five minutes, four times a week. She was also given a diet plan of low cholesterol, low carbohydrate, and less refined sugars with portion control. She was told to keep a daily log of her exercise and diet.

After four weeks, she reported that her mood had improved, and she was beginning to feel better. On her three-month visit, she was more talkative, engaging, and had started to lose weight. She also reported improved personal relationships with her friends and family. She had even started dating again, which she reported she hadn't done for years. On her six-month visit, she was totally in control of her life again and reported that it was the best she had felt in over a decade. She got a high-level job, and she had plans of writing a book. This shows that exercise and nutrition interventions can bring additional benefits to individuals who may already be taking antidepressants.[19]

Sleep and Rest

My next recommendations in the area of balancing your biochemistry for healing from depression are sleep and rest. Adequate sleep is generally considered to be about eight hours of restful sleep in every twenty-four-hour time period. This, along with regularly scheduled short periods of rest, are essential for emotional healing. Most people with depression are either sleeping excessively or not getting adequate sleep. If any of these describes you, you might want to pay attention to your sleep hygiene.

Sleep hygiene is a term used to describe all the practices that go into your sleeping routine. It covers issues such as your sleeping environment, the timing of your sleep, your daytime activities, and your diet. For a good mental and emotional wellbeing, it is important to have a regular routine, such as going to bed around the same time, engaging in almost the same preparatory activities before going to bed, refraining from using your bedroom for other activities such as watching TV or working on a computer, limiting exposure to bright lights especially from electronic devices and harsh temperatures while sleeping, limiting the intake of caffeine or spicy foods close to bedtime, and remaining physically active during the day.

Just like sleep, intentionally planned, regularly scheduled periods of rest can greatly enhance your emotional health. Contemporary society is fast-paced and stressful. We are burning the candle on both ends. Many people erroneously think that our productivity lies in how hard we work and how long we keep going without stopping. On the contrary, optimum productivity comes from hard work that is interspaced with regular rest times. Again, rest must be planned and regularly scheduled in order to be effective.

Antidepressant Medications

I have met a countless number of people, who want to heal from depression naturally without taking antidepressant medications. That sounds great, and many of us would go for any healing method that is efficacious without medications. The most-cited reasons for this rather widespread apprehension are the possibility of experiencing side effects, the possibility of having long-term adverse effects, and a dislike for the seemingly predatory disposition of the companies that produce these drugs. I also believe that Western society has become over-reliant on pharmacological products as a treatment method of choice. However, whoever is treading the road of healing-without-medications must do so cautiously.

Antidepressant medications do have an authoritative place in the treatment of depression. Antidepressants have proven effective to an appreciative extent in relieving the symptoms of depression. A recent large and comprehensive study on the efficacy of twenty-one antidepressants concluded that antidepressants are more effective than placebo in the acute treatment of adults with major depressive disorder.[20] A lot depends on the kind and severity of depression we are talking about. Depression may fall anywhere on a wide spectrum of moods depending on the cause and the severity.

One kind of depression is the brief sadness that results from the disappointment we experience when something does not go well for us. This may subside as soon as the offending situation resolves. Another kind of depression is the severe sense of loss, grief, anger, and/or despondency that results from suffering a break-up of an intimate relationship, losing a job, or losing a loved one prematurely. There is also a lingering sense of doom and anger that haunts you daily because of past trauma, multiple tragedies, unaccomplished dreams that have colored one's life. Finally, we have mild to severe depression that cannot be explained by any life situation—this kind can only be attributed to genetic, purely biological, or spiritual causes.

The decision to initiate or not initiate antidepressant medications will also depend on how severe your symptoms are and your likelihood of experiencing adverse outcomes. The potential negative outcomes from depression, which are too numerous to list, may include the loss of important relationships, reduced ability to function and be productive, and safety concerns including the risk to your life or the lives of others. In other words, if your depression is severe, is costing you a lot, and/or is likely to result in other significant losses, then a case should be made for antidepressant medications despite their potential side effects.

Least Effective Dosing

In my practice, I constantly compare the risks and benefits of placing my patients on antidepressants in order to make a decision that is in the best interest of the individual. Whenever I decide to prescribe antidepressants, I operate by the principle of least effective dosing. This means that there is no need for a higher dose if a lower dose is working just fine, and there is no need for an additional medication if the current number of medications is working just fine.

Again, if you are doing fairly well without antidepressants, I would often recommend non-medication interventions, such as psychotherapy or lifestyle modifications. With that said, I have witnessed multiple unfortunate situations where people shy away from antidepressants until they find themselves in psychiatric emergency centers needing crisis intervention. On the other hand, I have seen, in my practice, countless people experience night-and-day benefits from taking antidepressants. Tom (below) is just one of these beneficiaries.

"I Have Even Forgotten What It Feels like to Be Depressed."

Tom is a retired corporate executive in his mid-sixties. He was a high-achiever and was successful in his career but lost his drive for life. He lives at home with his wife. The couple has two adult children who live on their own. Tom came to see me for help with a deep and chronic depression that did not go away and did not respond to any treatment offered in the past several years. He came to me after his previous psychiatrist retired. He sought help from the Crisis Response Center as he thought of taking his life at one point. He is a nutrition and exercise fanatic who eats healthy and well-planned diets, does forty minutes of aerobic exercise daily, plus strength training three times a week.

Volunteering in the community interested him, but he could not get around to it. He has had insomnia most of his life. He constantly searched scientific journals for evidence-based treatments for depression.

After I completed my initial evaluation, we both agreed that we would focus more on medication interventions as he appeared to be paying close attention to the other areas of his life, including spirituality and meditation. For the first three months, we went through two failed antidepressant trials. Then I decided to add a bedtime dose of fifty milligrams of Quetiapine to his existing morning dose of twenty milligrams of Escitalopram daily. This combination became his magic potion. The addition of an atypical antipsychotic (Quetiapine, in this case) to an antidepressant (Escitalopram, in this case) as an adjunctive therapy for the treatment of major depressive disorder is a common practice among psychiatric practitioners. Tom's turnaround, however, was simply magical.

Recently, Tom reported to me that he has not experienced any symptom of depression for over one year now. He said, "Dr. Joy, I can't believe it. I have even forgotten what it feels like to be depressed." He is now sleeping well too. As you can imagine, Tom is now a self-styled expert in this area. He now brings me journal articles that show evidence for this line of treatment. This is an example of how an individual can derive tremendous benefits from the use of psychotropic medications when used alongside with non-medication interventions. A truly holistic healing approach will also consider Western medication at some level.

Complementary, Alternative, and Other Interventions

Several other treatment approaches are used to treat depression. The term "complementary and alternative interventions" is used to describe the group of interventions that are different from conventional medicine. When they are used in addition to conventional medicine, they are described as complementary, and when they are used instead of conventional medicine, they are described as alternative interventions. They include acupuncture, aromatherapy, diet and nutrition, dietary supplements, herbal medicine, light therapy, massage therapy, meditation, prayer, physical exercise, reiki, sound and music therapy, touch therapy, and yoga.[21] These, as well as transcranial magnetic stimulation (TMS), electroconvulsive therapy (ECT), and biofeedback have their place in the treatment of depression. I utilize or refer my patients to leverage several of these approaches in my treatment plans on a case-by-case basis with great success.

St. John's wort, dosed between 900 and 1,800 milligrams, is a popular herbal supplement used to relieve depression. It has been found to have antidepressant effects that are comparable to Selective Serotonin Reuptake Inhibitors (SSRIs—discussed ahead) for people who have mild to moderate depression.[22]

On a cautionary note, I have witnessed situations in which over-reliance on unregulated amounts or combinations of natural remedies resulted in cardiac and other life-threatening situations. This is because while natural remedies (such as St. John's wort, Omega-3 fatty acids, and S-adenosyl-L-methionine, SAMe) may appear to be generally healthier than Western pharmaceutical products, natural remedies also contain chemicals that can produce adverse health outcomes or interact negatively with other medications. Since they are not regulated or monitored by the Food and Drugs Administration (FDA), the onus lies on you to research what you are taking sufficiently or work with a provider who understands them. As you can see, in order to find a lasting treatment for depression, you need to be open-minded, intentional, integrated, and work with experts in the field.

Nutritional Supplements

Despite the cautionary note above, nutritional supplements such as vitamins and minerals are known to add great value to your mental health and your mood. This is because the average person struggles to maintain an adequately balanced diet. Dietary supplementation of Omega-3 fatty acid found in fish such as salmon and anchovies, Vitamins B and D, SAMe, Folic acid, and Magnesium have each been found to help boost neurotransmitter levels especially when taken in conjunction with antidepressants. In our technological age, the average person spends more time indoors than previous generations, and this puts us in danger of becoming vitamin D deficient. It is important to discuss dietary supplements with your medical provider for more individualized recommendations.

Examples of Antidepressants
- Selective Serotonin Reuptake Inhibitors (SSRIs), namely Fluoxetine (Prozac), Escitalopram (Lexapro), Sertraline, (Zoloft), Citalopram (Celexa), Paroxetine (Paxil), and Fluvoxamine (Luvox).

- Serotonin and Norepinephrine Reuptake Inhibitors (SNRIs) such as Duloxetine (Cymbalta), Venlafaxine (Effexor).
- Norepinephrine and dopamine reuptake inhibitors (NDRIs), such as Bupropion (Wellbutrin).
- Tricyclic Antidepressants (TCAs) such as Amitriptyline (Elavil) and Nortriptyline (Pamelor.
- Monoamine Oxidase Inhibitors (MAOIs) such as Selegeline.
- Noradrenergic and Specific Serotonergic Antidepressant (NASSA) such as Mirtazapine (Remeron).

Key Points for Antidepressant Use

- You need to take your antidepressant regularly whether you feel symptoms or not, as most antidepressants need to build up over time in order to be effective.
- When they work, antidepressants usually provide a general "upliftment" of mood or brighter outlook on life within 4-6 weeks after you start taking one.
- Antidepressants do not change your personality as some people think. They are meant to alter your mood.
- Unless otherwise advised by your prescriber, take antidepressants in the morning with food and a full glass of water.
- You do not have to remain on your antidepressant for life. Once you have been well for a reasonable period of time, you can work with your provider toward discontinuing your medication.

Discontinuation

If you feel like discontinuing your medication for any reason (whether it has stopped working, you are experiencing side effects, et cetera), wait and discuss this with your prescriber (except you are experiencing a severe reaction in which case you may stop immediately and notify your prescriber).

Common Side Effects of Antidepressants and How to Manage Them

- Headache: Drink a lot of water, get adequate rest, and consider taking over the-counter pain medications.
- Nausea: Eat smaller meals, sip ginger ale occasionally, consider taking an antacid.
- Dizziness: Drink a lot of water, rise/stand up slowly each time, consider taking medication at bedtime if does not interfere with your sleep.
- Dry mouth: Suck on ice chips or sugar-free hard candy, chew sugar-free gum.
- Sexual side effects (Reduced sexual desire, delayed organism, erectile dysfunction): Discuss options with your partner; schedule sexual activity before taking medication; have your partner initiate sexual activity; improve sexual practices, e.g. Put more effort into foreplay.
- Weight gain: Schedule mealtimes, eat healthy meals, exercise regularly, and track your weight over time.
- Weight loss: Schedule mealtimes, make meals more appetizing, choose higher- calorie meals (e.g. peanut butter and banana), track your weight over a period

of time, consider flavoring your food, consider protein supplements, see a dietician.

- Diarrhea: Drink a lot of water, consider Gatorade to replenish electrolytes.
- Constipation: Drink a lot of water, eat high-fiber foods, increase physical activity, and consider stool softeners, discuss with your doctor.
- Suicidal Ideation: Call your doctor, seek emergency care as soon as possible.
- Excessive activation/Elevation of Mood: Discuss with prescriber as further evaluation may be needed for Bipolar disorder.

Always discuss the benefits versus side effects with your prescriber. Your prescriber may consider a slow-release formulation or switching to another agent.

Chapter 6

The Spiritual Dimension

"Man is a spirit, he has a soul, and he lives in a body."
– Kenneth E. Hagin

Have you ever thought about who you truly are? I hope so! There is far more to you than meets the eye. The spiritual dimension of the Authentic Healing Process for Depression (AHPD) is based on the foundation that you and I are primarily spiritual entities. This is true because the scripture says in Genesis 1:26-27 that God made us in His image. If God is spirit (John 4:24) and He made us in His image, then we must be spiritual beings. Do not ignore this fundamental truth because it is a key to receiving lasting healing from any form of illness that you may experience in your life. Your body is only your housing or "container," that is, the part of you that helps you to live here on earth. Your mind, your will, and your emotions make up your soul. Your spirit and your soul are closely intertwined, and they constitute your inner parts.

Knowing that man is primarily a spiritual entity, you will agree with me that real and lasting healing cannot focus narrowly on the body alone. Sustainable change in any area of our lives can only happen when it begins on the inside of us. Similarly, authentic healing can only occur when your inner parts are healed as well. Jesus Christ made this very clear when He said in Matthew 23:26, *"Blind Pharisee, first cleanse the inside of the cup and dish, that the outside of them may be clean also."* It is sad to note that some of our clinical interventions are rather cosmetic. They fail to address the core of the problem—our inner parts.

Spirituality

The spiritual dimension of the AHPD has a lot to offer you. I pray that you do not underestimate the power in the spiritual resources that are available to you in your journey from depression to victory. Simply put, spirituality is your connectedness with your source. A spiritual person is one who is closely connected with his or her origin. To be truly spiritual is to be in sync with your source. To be spiritual is to be plugged into "something" way bigger than yourself, which is your source of being and your source of sustenance. What do I mean by source? Your source is where you come from—not your hometown, not your ancestry, but how you came to be on earth and how you came to be borne by your parents. Your source is the entity that holds your life in place. According to Acts 17:28, *"...for in Him we live and move and have our being, as also some of your own poets have said, for we are also His offspring."* Dear friend, God is your source! Once you are plugged into Him, you can be sure that your well will never run dry.

The Role of Source and Destiny in Emotional Healing

Once you discover and reconnect with where you come from, you need to understand where you are going from there— your destiny. These two discoveries will initiate a series of transformational processes and "Aha" moments in your life. These revelations will help you to tap into the vast spiritual resources that are available to expedite your journey out of depression into a place of true joy and fulfillment in life. Friend, there is nothing as powerful as the illuminating and liberating power of knowledge and revelation! Often, the ability of a captain to clearly identify his geographical coordinates can be a source of relief to a ship that is in distress. As humans, we draw strength from our source, and we are motivated by our destiny. These two revelations provide us with our spiritual coordinates.

The Role of Answers to the Fundamental Questions of Life

The late Dr. Myles Munroe told a phenomenal story about how he came to answer the two questions above (Where do I come from? Where am I going from here?), as well as three other fundamental questions of life: Who am I? Why am I here? What can I do? He was a thirteen-year-old boy growing up in an impoverished part of the Bahamas. His father was a pastor who preached that God loved man and wanted the best for man. However, little Myles and his family's realities did not reflect what his father preached. Despite their faith in God, they lived a life of depravity. Little Myles decided to embark on a mission to find answers to the questions above. He went to the most popular and most widely circulated book of all time, the Holy Bible. Of course, if you had a shot at the best place to find answers to such serious questions of life, wouldn't you go to the most credible book on the planet? He began to read, memorize, and meditate on portions of the Bible, starting from the gospel of John. What happened was simply mind-blowing! He found the answers that he was looking for, and he experienced a 180-degree, inside-out transformation in his life as a result. He lived the rest of his life empowering individuals, leaders, groups, and nations to experience the kind of illumination, healing, and transformation that he experienced.

From Discouraged to Joy-Filled

I can proudly say that I am one of the individuals whose lives have been transformed by the ministry of the late Dr. Munroe. As a teenager, he discovered that God needs man to establish His kingdom on earth. Similarly, Satan needs man in order to accomplish his agenda on earth. This is because spirits without physical bodies cannot function on earth. In other words, there is an ongoing spiritual battle for our bodies. For this reason, God is not only interested in your healing and general wellbeing; He is heavily invested in your healing! Once Dr. Munroe understood this truth, the spirit of God literally came alive within him, and he became transformed from a perplexed and discouraged boy into a confident and joy-filled young man, full of faith and fearless audacity. No wonder he lived all his life empowered and also empowered millions in his lifetime. I pray that this will be your story as well.

When you look at the ultra-intelligence that is displayed by nature, you cannot deny that there must be an architect at work behind the scenes. Consider the human body and the intricate and expert nature in which our organ systems, organs, and tissues have been and put together and made to function. Consider that your heart beats 40 million times each year, that you have lived on earth without any effort on your part to keep your body systems working. Creation is simply a supernatural masterpiece! And every masterpiece must have a mastermind behind it. This must communicate to us that no human being is an accident. Yes, you are not an accident. You did not just come to exist. You are a masterpiece designed by God for a unique purpose. No human was born empty. You are equipped with all that it takes to deliver on your purpose. You also have an obligation to give a report to your Maker on what you did here on earth in relation to what you were destined to do.

God Wants You Healed

I have good news for you! God, your Creator, is interested in your health and healing. Because He made you for a purpose, He is interested in your healing even more than you might be. Because of that, He has provided a way for you to be healed. God wants you healed—totally! God wants you healed bodily, emotionally, and spiritually. He made provision for your healing in His Son Jesus Christ. According to John 3:16 (New King

James Version), "."*For God so loved the world that He gave His only begotten Son, that whoever believes in Him should not perish but have everlasting life*

When Jesus came to the earth, He boldly declared part of his mission on earth as follows. Luke 4:18-19, "*The Spirit of the Lord is upon me, because He has anointed me to preach the gospel to the poor; He has sent me to heal the brokenhearted, to proclaim liberty to the captives, and recovery of sight to the blind, to set at liberty those who are oppressed; to proclaim the acceptable year of the Lord.*"

There you have it! In John 3:16, God made provision for your salvation and spiritual healing. In Luke 4:18-19, God made provision for your emotional healing. The way to activate this healing is to read God's Word for yourself, genuinely believe what it says without doubting, confess with your mouth what you believed, and act according to your belief and confession without wavering. I hope you are saying to yourself right now, "This seems so simple. I can totally do this!" Yes, it may seem simple, but it is also exceedingly profound and life-transforming. The sad reality is that, despite being simple and despite being profound, many have failed to tap into these rich spiritual resources. I pray that you will not fall prey to this deception. Take a moment and practice the above.

Start a New Journey with God

You know what? God is not interested in your healing only. He is even more interested in your destiny and in having a relationship with you. I urge you to begin your spiritual walk with God today. I need you to know that you should not follow God only because you want to be healed by Him. We do not follow

God for what we can get from Him. We follow God, obey Him, and serve Him because He is God, our Maker, and we love Him. Guess what happens? God in turn blesses us with what we need.

Pray the following prayer to God slowly and genuinely and believe in your heart that God will hear you and grant your request: *"Heavenly Father, I believe in your Son Jesus Christ, and I invite Him to be my Lord and my Master. I am sorry for living my life my own way thereby sinning against you. I confess my shortcomings, and I submit myself to your will. Please forgive my sins and accept me as your child. Help me to spend eternity with you. Thank you for answering my prayer today, amen!"*

When genuinely offered, this is the kind of prayer that helps to establish or re-establish your spiritual connection with your source. Taking this bold step positions you in a place where you can enjoy all that God provides to His children. Becoming a child of God alone is an essential part of your healing and probably more important than the emotional healing you might be looking for. After all, what would your life amount to if your depression gets cured, but your soul gets lost? The following scripture captures this so well, *"…For what profit is it to a man if he gains the whole world, and is himself destroyed or lost?"* (Luke 9:25).

Your relationship with God needs to be maintained on an ongoing basis through the reading and studying of the Bible, meeting and sharing fellowship with other Christians, praying regularly, and sharing your faith with others. If there is one thing you should remember, it is the fact that God loves you dearly and wants to maintain an ongoing father-child love relationship with you. He wants to envelop you with the warmth of His embrace, and He wants you to find shelter in His mighty arms. If depression looms in the horizon, it is comforting to know that God has promised in His word never to leave you or forsake you (Hebrews 13:5) and that you will outlive your challenges and not be destroyed (Isaiah 43:2) when you walk closely with Him.

Guilt Melts Away

Blanca is a fifty-eight-year old law-enforcement officer who recently came to see me at my clinic for the first time after several years of seeing multiple psychiatric providers. One of her previous doctors had prescribed 150 mg of Sertraline once daily for the treatment of depression and anxiety for a period of five years. She rated both her depression and anxiety as moderate on a scale of mild to severe. She informed her provider that she had a "horrible" past, which she is currently paying for. As a teenager, she had terminated several pregnancies as she was promiscuous and not ready to have children but failed to use protection.

Blanca said to me, "Doctor, I am a basket case! Several times a day, I see the dark shadow of a huge man standing by me. He is so huge I can see only his feet. I hear this man pointing me to a large group of children who are constantly crying and telling the man to punish me." She would experience panic attacks from time to time as a result of these experiences. She also had nightmares, insomnia, and did not like quiet areas as the voices became worse when it was quiet. She understood this to mean, "The babies I killed are asking God for revenge. God will never forgive me!" I increased her Sertraline to 200 mg daily and started Christian cognitive behavioral therapy, which was Blanca's preference. I added Clonazepam 0.5 mg once daily as needed to help with her anxiety for a short period of time. Targeted Bible study, affirmations, prayers, and meditation featured prominently in her treatment. After six months of using these spiritual interventions, she returned to me with a broad affect, relaxed posture, and a bright mood with only mild anxiety that did not interfere with her functioning. She no longer had depression and her guilt and hallucinations greatly reduced in intensity and frequency. She is currently extremely happy about her turnaround, and she understands that she needs to continue with these interventions as a lifestyle. The healing embedded in the power of God is a treasure that is yet to be discovered by many.

A Sample Prayer for Healing

When you establish a genuine loving relationship with God, you will soon realize that you are up to something phenomenal. You can come boldly to God because He is your Father and He is invested in your wellbeing! You can ask Him to heal any impairment in your mood. Ask God to heal the depression and anxiety that afflict you and ask him to plant His joy in your heart. While doing this, you must believe that God has healed you. When you are ready, say the following prayer genuinely, believing that God will heal you: *"Father God, you made me, and I know you are willing and able to heal me. Your Word says in III John verse 2 that You want me to be healed. Lord, please heal me and give me permanent victory over depression and anxiety in the name of your Son Jesus Christ. Based on your word, I declare that I am healed. Thank you for my healing! Amen!"* After a prayer like this one, you must continue to thank God for as long as you live, that you are healed and hold onto your faith without wavering.

Forgive Yourself and Forgive Others

Now that God has forgiven and healed you, it is important that you forgive yourself and anyone that has offended you. One of the major symptoms of depression is guilt. Guilt makes you more self-blaming than you should be. For instance, guilt will whisper into your ears repeatedly, "You indeed brought this depression upon yourself! You remember when you lived a reckless life in your teenage years? You must have harmed many people in the process! Karma is real! It is payback time!" On the other hand, you might have been offended by someone in the past, which may have left an emotional wound in your heart. Unresolved bitterness is a canker that will eat you up to the core if not promptly dealt with. This is a good time to forgive and release others for your own sake. Bitterness and unforgiveness are often implicated in or perpetuators of depressed mood. As you embark on your spiritual journey, I need you to know that it takes a heart conviction, a genuine decision, a simple but fervent prayer, and a lifestyle change that reflects your convictions for this to work for you.

Friend, the Bible is a healing powerhouse. If you are not yet leveraging this powerful resource, I urge you to begin now. A core component of your new journey with God is to read a portion of the Bible on a daily basis. There are devotional books (such as *Living Word* by Dr. Mensa Otabil and *Our Daily Bread*) that will guide you through this process so that you would not be overwhelmed. Beyond your daily reading, you also need to intentionally affirm carefully selected healing-related scriptures as part of your journey to victory. There is tremendous power in declaring the word of God over your situation. When this is done consistently and in faith, your confession will eventually become your possession. I cannot emphasize to you enough the healing properties of the Holy Scriptures. I have included some healing scriptures and affirmations below to help you get started. Dare to read the Bible. Believe it. Confess it. Put it into action and see the results for yourself. One scripture a day may be literally as effective as one pill a day in your healing process. Imagine what a combination of these two resources can do! That is the philosophy behind the AHPD.

Are Medications Anti-Christian?

A patient once said to me, "Doctor, I told my pastor that you prescribe medications for my depression, and he was very shocked. He wondered why you prescribe medications when you're a pastor." This is a deception in a segment of our society today—the erroneous thinking that faith and science do not mix. My answer to that is two other questions: "Who made the herbs used to produce medications? Who gave wisdom and ability to the people who formulated and manufactured the medications?" The resounding answer to both questions is God! So, if God made the herbs and granted the resources for medications to be produced, why should the people of God avoid something that was granted by God?

Another set of items in our healing toolbox is prayer and meditation. Friend, I encourage you to leverage the benefits of prayer and spiritual meditation in your healing process. Prayer is communication with God. You can pray to God as regularly as you talk to others around you. Perhaps the most illustrative scripture about prayer in the Bible is Matthew 7:7, "*Ask, and it will be given to you; seek, and you will find; knock, and it will be opened to you.*" Isn't this awesome? This is what I call a blank check. When you pray, have faith that God will heal you, and I believe He will (See Mark 11:22). I do not know how He will heal you, and I do not know when He will heal you, but I know He heals. Many people cannot wrap their minds around this because it is a spiritual concept, and spiritual things only make sense to spiritual people (See 1 Corinthians 2:14). After all, what do you have to lose when you pray? However, you have a lifetime of healing to gain.

Having done that, is it possible that God will not heal you? Yes. Although God is a million times able to Heal, He is not obligated to heal, and we must not presume that He will heal us. He may have a bigger purpose for your pain. In some situations, instead of removing our challenges, God chooses to strengthen us so we can endure our challenges (Read 2 Corinthians 12:7-9). According to Isaiah 40:31, "*But those who wait on the Lord shall renew their strength; They shall mount up with wings like eagles. They shall run and not be weary. They shall walk and not faint.*" May God renew your strength as you wait upon Him in total confidence and obedient trust. Please note that waiting upon the Lord is being used in an active sense. It is not referring to being dormant or literally sitting down and expecting a miracle. It means having total dependence, absolute trust, and permanent confidence that God will deliver. It means to have rest and a blessed assurance in God.

A Lifestyle of Prayer

Friend, prayer does bring tremendous results! Prayer may be intercessory, personal, or corporate in nature. Intercessory prayer is when others pray for you. While this works, do not rely only on others to pray for you. You should engage in personal prayer because each one of us has direct access to God. Corporate prayer, where a number of people agree and pray about a situation, also generates tremendous results. Oh, how I wish that you would *taste and see* that the Lord is indeed good (Psalm 34:8)! As you start the incredible lifestyle of prayer, I need you to know that one of the methods of prayer that I have seen working every single time is the P.U.S.H. method, which stands for "Pray Until Something Happens!" I guess that is self-explanatory.

Christian meditation is when you cut off all distraction momentarily and focus solely on a portion of scripture and ruminate on it over and over again until you receive a deeper revelation and strength or healing from it. And if you knew anything about revelation—revelation is the trigger for or the doorway to transformation. In his book, *The Purpose Driven Life (Zondervan),* Rick Warren states, "No other habit can do more to transform your life and make you more like Jesus than daily reflection on Scripture... If you look up all the times God speaks about meditation in the Bible, you will be amazed at the benefits He has promised to those who take the time to reflect on His Word throughout the day." God gives perfect peace to those whose minds are continually focused on Him (Isaiah 26:3).

Developing and maintaining an eternal perspective to living is a great tool for fulfillment in life. When you know that your life counts for more than what we currently see and that there is more to life than the time we spend on the earth, you became motivated to keep persevering. This is one of the core concepts of the AHPD. It is the reason that the AHPD is presented as a never-ending wheel. In other words, it is not over until God says it is over. It is because of an eternal perspective that we never give up in the game of life. An eternal perspective is what makes us want to live right. We endeavor to live right because we know there are rewards and penalties for what we do on earth. An eternal perspective motivates me to die empty, that is, to die after I have deployed all that is within me.

The reason some people get discouraged and never heal from depression is that they have lost focus on the eternal. They have lost focus on the heavenly goal. God wants us to maintain our focus on Him rather than on our suffering (See Colossians 3:2). People who lack an eternal perspective are prone to thinking that it is over for them because they are in pain and their lives are threatened. Friend, even in the presence of your symptoms, God has promised to give you rest when you come to Him (Matthew 11:28). Yes, you can enjoy the rest that God gives. There is a peace that permeates through the storms of our lives and it can only come from God.

Your Life Is Not Over

It is a deception to think that your life is over only because you are afflicted by an illness such as depression. Depression is not a life sentence. If you have not yet completed your assignment on earth, then tighten your belt because it is not likely that your life will be over soon. Even death is not final, let alone a life of troubles. A good way to see the AHPD, therefore is to understand it as a lifestyle concept rather than a mere depression treatment approach. What I am advocating is more of lifestyle modification than a one-time intervention in your life. Remember that you will never complete traveling along the Authentic Healing Wheel (Fig. 1).

Practicing Joy Is a Game-Changer

Two additional spiritual interventions that are effective for healing depression are practicing joy and practicing kindness. Practicing joy is based on the Apostle Paul's instruction in Philippians 4:4 "*Rejoice in the Lord always. Again, I will say, rejoice!*" Our happiness is dependent on circumstances, but our joy is not. While something good must be happening in order for you to be happy, nothing good needs to be happening in order for you to rejoice. Joy is a conscious and unconditional decision and it must come from deep within your heart. In Philippians 4:4, Apostle Paul is implying that rejoicing is completely under your control. You should see me—I am already bubbling with joy as I write this. I know you feel depressed. I know you don't feel like rejoicing. I know you are feeling down, but this has nothing to do with how you are feeling. Right now, pause reading for a moment and laugh out loud! Dance if you can! Shout to yourself, "I choose to rejoice in the Lord no matter how I feel!" Maybe you're in public, and you don't want to be seen as a weird person. I totally understand! If so, just let out a broad smile for no reason and whisper to yourself, "I choose to rejoice in the Lord always."

You see, practicing joy is not only a spiritual intervention; it is also a psychological tool and a biochemical intervention. You obey the Word of God when you practice joy. You send chemical signals to your brain, telling your brain to operate in joy mode when you practice joy. You're programming yourself for joy when you practice joy. Will it seem odd? Oh yes! Will it seem fake? Yes, it will! Why do something that seems both odd and fake? Because the Word of God says so and because it works! Every morning when you wake up, declare to yourself, "*This is the day the Lord has made; [I] will rejoice and be glad in it*" (Psalm 118:24). When you do this habitually, before long, your confession will become your possession, and your obedience to the Word of God will produce tremendous results.

Practicing kindness is another game-changer. This is a lifestyle choice that defies the odds and propels you to reach over to do for others what you are in need of yourself. Isn't this awesome? This is what makes a person who is depressed put a smile on the faces of others. You may deliberately practice kindness by saying a kind word to someone such as, "You look so beautiful!" You may practice kindness by holding the door open for someone. You may practice kindness by listening patiently while someone shares his or her frustrations. The list is endless. Beware that this has to be deliberate. It will not come to you naturally. However, there is an inherent reciprocal healing virtue in this course of action. You have to experience it in order to know how it feels.

Practicing gratitude is a powerful way to lift your mood and heal from depression. The timeless Christian hymn[23] tells us that when you have heavy burdens and discouragements, and you are thinking that all is lost, one way to keep yourself singing as the days go by is to count your blessings and name them one by one. You legitimately have a lot to worry about. But wait! Let's start by being grateful that your heart is beating, that you can breathe, and that you can read this book. Why not add this to your daily routine? Thank God for a newborn day, the sunshine, the air you breathe, and birds that sing away, and the deep blue sea as Jim Reeves admonishes. This is one activity that you can be proactive and deliberate about every morning. You should see me as I type—I am singing as my day goes by. Before long, you will also be singing as the days go by!

Many Have Traveled This Road

Looking through the scriptures, we see many giants of the faith who felt emotionally down, some to the point of being depressed at some point in their lives. Each of them, however, overcame through some of the same principles discussed in this book. Job suffered devastating losses and a debilitating illness. His unflinching faith in God and the company of his three friends helped him to bounce back. Whenever you're feeling down, surround yourself with good friends. The Prophet Elijah, who could stop the rain from falling on earth for three and a half years, became so depressed that he asked God to take his life. Elijah survived depression because he rested. He was nourished when an angel brought him food and water. He found a new mission to continue serving the Lord, and God gave him an assistant by the name Elisha to be his companion and helper. Jeremiah was so depressed that he wrote a whole book called Lamentations. He, however, survived by feeding on God's word. He said in Jeremiah 15:16, "*Your words were found, and I ate them, And Your word was to me the joy and rejoicing of my heart...*"

King David, who was a friend of God, was severely emotionally distressed when all the men around him turned against him and threatened to kill him. The Bible says in 1 Samuel 30:6 that

David encouraged himself in the Lord. The way to encourage yourself in the Lord and jumpstart your healing is to personalize and repeatedly confess the word of God. See below for some suggestions for daily affirmations. Our Lord Jesus Christ Himself was described as "… *A man of sorrows and acquainted with grief…*" (Isaiah 53:3). At one point in the Garden of Gethsemane, He told his disciples, "… *My soul is exceedingly sorrowful, even to death…*" (Matthew 26:38). How did he survive his sorrows? He yielded Himself totally to His Father's will and prayed His way through the darkest moments of His life (remember P.U.S.H.?). If you would apply yourself to the biblical solutions outlined above, I have no doubt that the light of God will break through the dark moments of your life and bring you joy like never before. Remember, "… *Weeping may endure for a night, but joy comes in the morning*" (Psalm 30:5).

Christian Affirmations for Healing

The following are examples of Bible-based affirmations. Feel free and use them as often as you can. The scriptural bases are provided in parentheses. Read them aloud as many times are you need to. Remember that these are not just mere words. John 6:63 tells us that the Words of God are spirit and they are life. The Holy Spirit will come upon you and heal every ailment in your body as you make these confessions by faith.

Healing Affirmation 1

I believe in God, and I believe in the power of His Word.

The Word of God says that God wants me to be healed (3 John 2).

The Word of God also says that my words have the power to shape my life (Proverbs 18:20-21).

By faith, I declare that I am healed in Jesus's mighty name!

In the name of Jesus, I terminate and reject depression right now! I reject anxiety! I put them behind me forever.

I will no longer be sad because the joy of the Lord is my strength (Nehemiah 8:10).

This is the day the Lord the Lord has made. I will rejoice and be glad in it (Psalm 118:24).

No matter how low I feel right now, I know that I am more than a conqueror through Christ who loves me (Romans 8:37).

My healing is complete in Jesus Christ. I seal my healing by the blood of Jesus.

In Jesus's mighty name! Amen!

Healing Affirmation 2

I believe that Jesus is the Son of God and I know that He is alive.

When Jesus was on earth, He healed every sick person that was brought to Him (Matthew 4:23-24).

While He was on the cross, He declared that "It is finished!" (John 19:30)

Jesus paid a full price for my healing.

He took my infirmities and bore my sicknesses (Matthew 8:17).

Therefore, I will not be afflicted with depression anymore.

By His stripes, I am healed! (Isaiah 53:5)

My God promised in His Word that He would not leave me or forsake me.

He said in His word that, even though I may go through the valley of the shadow of death, He will be with me and He will comfort me. I receive comfort from God's presence today! (Psalm 23:4)

By faith, I dismiss depression now! It is now a thing of the past.

My mind is at peace. My heart will rejoice in the Lord forever. Amen!

Healing Affirmation 3

I am a child of God (John 1:12).

I know that sickness does not come from God, so my depression is not of God.

Jesus said that anything that is not planted by God will be uprooted (Matthew 15:13-14).

Jesus also said that because I have faith, I will say to this mountain of depression, 'Move from here to there,' and it will move; and nothing will be impossible for me (Matthew 17:20).

In Exodus 15:26, my God has promised that He is the Lord who heals me.

On this basis, I exercise the healing power of God upon my life today.

I command the chemicals in my brain to come into a healthy balance.

I command new brain cells to be produced and my brain cells to come alive now.

I command my mind to become joyful and my body to become vibrant.

I decree and I declare that I have total healing from depression. I pronounce that I am depression-free!

I command the elements of the universe—the sun, the mood, and the stars—to work in my favor.

As I pursue my purpose in life, take my medications, I engage in therapy, I connect with others, I engage in physical exercise, and I eat a healthy diet;

As I love God and my neighbor, I command that all things will work together for my good and bring me total healing (Romans 8:28).

I am totally and permanently healed from depression.

In the name of Jesus Christ my Savior! Amen!

Affirmations for a Sound Sleep

By faith, I decree that I do not have problems sleeping anymore.

As I lay my head down to sleep, my thoughts are calm, and my body is peaceful.

I will sleep well tonight, and I will be well-rested in the morning.

This is because my God gives His beloved sleep (Psalm 127:2).

He said that He has given me His peace, the peace that the world cannot give (John 14:27).

I have the peace of God that surpasses all understanding. The peace of God guards my heart and my mind (Philippians 4:7).

I am not afraid of any terror by night (Psalm 91:5).

My mind is at peace. Perfect peace.

Goodnight to me! In Jesus' name!

Ten Biblical Prescriptions for Emotional Healing

The following are a few scripture passages that relate to healing. Feel free to look them up and read, study, memorize, and confess as often as possible. Remember—God's words carry the power to transform your life.

Why are you cast down, O my soul? And why are you disquieted within me?

Hope in God, for I shall yet praise Him For the help of His countenance (Psalm 42:5).

Many are the afflictions of the righteous, But the Lord delivers him out of them all (Psalm 34:19).

Peace I leave with you, My peace I give to you; not as the world gives do I give to you. Let not your heart be troubled, neither let it be afraid. (John 14:27).

Bless the Lord, O my soul; and all that is within me, bless His holy name!

Bless the Lord, O my soul, and forget not all His benefits:

Who forgives all your iniquities, who heals all your diseases,

Who redeems your life from destruction, who crowns you with lovingkindness and tender mercies,

Who satisfies your mouth with good things, So that your youth is renewed like the eagle's (Psalm 103: 1-5).

Come to Me, all you who labor and are heavy laden, and I will give you rest (Matthew 11:28).

To console those who mourn in Zion, To give them beauty for ashes, The oil of joy for mourning, The garment of praise for the spirit of heaviness; That they may be called trees of righteousness, The planting of the Lord, that He may be glorified (Isaiah 61:3).

He who dwells in the secret place of the Most High shall abide under the shadow of the Almighty.

I will say of the Lord, "He is my refuge and my fortress; My God, in Him I will trust."

Surely He shall deliver you from the snare of the fowler and from the perilous pestilence.

He shall cover you with His feathers, and under His wings you shall take refuge;

His truth shall be your shield and buckler.

You shall not be afraid of the terror by night, nor of the arrow that flies by day,

Nor of the pestilence that walks in darkness, nor of the destruction that lays waste at noonday.

A thousand may fall at your side, and ten thousand at your right hand; But it shall not come near you.

Only with your eyes shall you look and see the reward of the wicked.

Because you have made the Lord, who is my refuge, Even the Most High, your dwelling place,

No evil shall befall you, nor shall any plague come near your dwelling;

For He shall give His angels charge over you, to keep you in all your ways.

In their hands they shall bear you up, lest you dash your foot against a stone.

You shall tread upon the lion and the cobra; The young lion and the serpent you shall trample underfoot.

"Because he has set his love upon Me, therefore I will deliver him; I will set him on high, because he has known My name.

He shall call upon Me, and I will answer him; I will be with him in trouble; I will deliver him and honor him.

With long life I will satisfy him and show him My salvation. (Psalm 91)

I will lift up my eyes to the hills—From whence comes my help?

My help comes from the Lord, who made heaven and earth.

He will not allow your foot to be moved; He who keeps you will not slumber.

Behold, He who keeps Israel Shall neither slumber nor sleep.

The Lord is your keeper; The Lord is your shade at your right hand.

The sun shall not strike you by day, nor the moon by night.

The Lord shall preserve you from all evil; He shall preserve your soul.

The Lord shall preserve your going out and your coming in from this time forth, and even forevermore. (Psalm 121).

And He said to me, "My grace is sufficient for you, for My strength is made perfect in weakness." Therefore most gladly I will rather boast in my infirmities, that the power of Christ may rest upon me.[10] Therefore I take pleasure in infirmities, in reproaches, in needs, in persecutions, in distresses, for Christ's sake. For when I am weak, then I am strong (2 Corinthians 12:9-10).

I waited patiently for the Lord; And He inclined to me and heard my cry.

He also brought me up out of a horrible pit, out of the miry clay, and set my feet upon a rock, and established my steps.

He has put a new song in my mouth—Praise to our God; Many will see it and fear, and will trust in the Lord (Psalm 40:1-3).

Chapter 7

The Social Dimension

"When we replace 'I' with 'We,'
'illness' becomes 'wellness.'"
– Anonymous

S ocial isolation is one of the major symptoms of depression. If you feel depressed, I bet you probably want to
be by yourself. You probably don't feel like going out or
hanging out, even in the company of people you love. You may
feel uncomfortable in public. This may be because you think
you have major defects that will be noticed by others. It may be
because you feel irritable and people tend to get on your nerves.
Sometimes, you just can't stand people. Depression convinces
you that you just like being alone. This is one of the weapons

that depression uses to destroy its victims. Social isolation has been associated with negative mental health outcomes in various segments of modern society.[24]

The popularity and overuse of social media has certainly not helped with this situation. While social media has helped to connect people from afar, it has threatened the development of genuine physical contact among families, friends, and neighbors. It has become commonplace to see family members in a car or in a room with each person talking or browsing on their phone instead of interacting with the others. Many in our society have become lonely while they may be in a room full of other people. Even when people connect, they only connect at a surface and casual level with no real, deep, genuine relationships or care for one another.

The Dangers of Isolation

While it is a good thing to create time that you can be alone for a purpose, there are many dangers associated with being alone. For instance, crimes and offenses are usually committed under the cover of darkness or when no one is looking. Being alone makes you feel powerless. The helplessness that you feel when you are alone can quickly develop into other adverse outcomes before you know it. The feeling of helplessness quickly escalates into despondency. Before you know it, you are convinced that you are "the only one that feels this way." Before you know it, you're telling yourself, "It is over for me. Things will never get better. I am done! There is nothing I can do." Before you know it, you're throwing in the towel. That is the power of isolation. It quickly erodes your confidence and dissipates your energy. If you're in that situation, please note that you are not alone. Many have traveled that route. However, you're not in the right place. It is a dangerous road to travel on. Don't stay on this road for a long time. It does not lead to a good place.

I know you don't feel like talking to or being in the company of others, but therein lies your power to heal. If you're going to heal from depression, you must factor other people into your healing process. There is an immense medicinal value in your connectedness to others. The more connected you are to others, the more likely you are to heal. Of course, this has to be done with wisdom. I am not saying you should go around telling everyone about your problems. I am not even saying that you should share company with anyone that comes around. Some relationships are rather toxic, and some people will drain you rather than help you. The point is that there is a tremendous emotional benefit in social connections.

The Striking Importance of Healthy Social Connections

In a major Harvard study on relationships called the Alameda County Study, a group of scientists led by social scientist George Kaplan Ph.D. followed 7,000 people over nine years and found that those who maintained meaningful social connections turned out to be healthier than those that ate healthy meals. Study participants who were the most isolated were three times more likely to die than those who maintained healthy relationships. The benefits of strong social connectedness were found to override the risks of poor health habits (This is not a license for unhealthy habits!). In reference to this study, American Author and Christian Minister John Ortberg indicated, "It is better to eat Twinkies with friends than to eat broccoli alone."

The Benefits of Withdrawing from a Toxic Relationship

My partner and I have been working with a male client in his early twenties for the past few years. An aunt and uncle raised him due to his parents being involved with drugs. After living with his aunt and uncle, the client moved in with his older brother. The client went to a therapist due to depression and anxiety that could not be fully controlled with medications. Upon further assessment, it became apparent that the client's only social connections were with his brother and his brother's friends. Obviously, the client felt somewhat isolated. He also reported almost every two weeks that he had a physical altercation with the brother, and on several occasions the police were called, sometimes by bystanders. The brother was a drug dealer, and the client reported that he often felt paranoid, "like I have to constantly look over my shoulder."

The therapist worked with the client as he made the change in his life of leaving his brother after four years and moving out on his own. He maintained a firm boundary between him and his brother. The stress of being around the illegal drug business was lifted, and the client's anxiety began to lift as well. The client then began establishing friendships and indeed reconnecting with friends he hadn't spoken to in years. The client's depression has also been alleviated as he moved out into the world on his own and made social connections. He has remained on depression and anxiety medications while making these changes.

The client now holds down a job, is doing better in school, and hopes to move up the professional ladder. Essential in the client's recovery progress was both drawing clear boundaries with his previous, toxic relationship and creating new social connections on his own terms.

Yes, You Have a Potential Support System

We all have people at various levels of closeness in our lives. Beware that depression will tell you that you don't have anyone in your life, but you need to know that depression is a big liar! It makes you believe in the weirdest lies ever. I once had an interesting exchange with one of my clients. He was going through multiple life stressors, including family drama with his teenage children becoming wayward, which was, in turn, tearing apart his marriage. He was also facing a major financial disaster, and he just heard the news from his doctor that he might have a rare and aggressive form of cancer.

While we talked, I tried to identify possible aspects of his support system, but he repeatedly and aggressively denied that there was anyone in his life who could help. I stated, "This is the time to open up to your wife and ask for her support." He responded, "She is busy working, and she does not have time." I added, "How about if you just tried. You might get her to listen, you know?" Then I added, "How about taking a day off work so you can attend to your health?" Shaking his head, he replied, "You don't even know what you're talking about. My boss doesn't even want to hear that. I will lose my job if I attempt that." This went on and on and on until I realized that it was no longer the actual person that was talking, but it was his depression that was talking for him.

By this time, you might have noticed that I hate depression. You're right—I hate depression with a passion, and I will do anything to defeat it and replace it with joy and fulfillment. Here are the reasons I hate depression: Just like the gentleman in the story above, depression eliminates your logic and makes you think in a negatively skewed way. Depression erodes your self-confidence and makes you feel extremely incapable of doing even the simplest things. Depression steals your joy from you and replaces it with fabricated sorrow that has no basis. The only paint in the closet of depression is black paint; it paints everything dark and essentially leaves you color-blind regarding anything good happening in your life. Depression can snatch your promise and your destiny. As you are well aware, depression has proven time and time again that it can end lives abruptly and cut off human life mercilessly.

See why I hate this monster called depression? I would like to recruit you to partner with me in the fight against depression. All you need to do is trust in the process and leverage it to any length possible in order to eliminate depression in your own life. If I can get you to become depression-free for life, I will be one of the happiest men on earth. Now, I am going to do something like what I did with the gentleman in my story above, and I hope that you know better than to repeat what he did.

Your Potential Supports

Coming back to your support system, you most likely have your close family and/or close friends who form your core network. Please say, "Yes." This may include your spouse, children, parents, siblings, your pastor or another spiritual leader, or friends. Then you have a second layer of people who may still be close to you but not close enough to belong to the core. Beyond this, you have acquaintances or people that you know only on a casual basis, maybe by name only. This third group may include your neighbors, your coworkers, fellow church/club members, et cetera. I hope that you can see through the dark and see the crowd of people around you. These people are only contacts at this time, but they are only a step away from becoming part of your support system.

If you're severely depressed or having thoughts of not wanting to be alive but you're not suicidal, you must talk to someone now. I recommend talking to your primary care doctor, your psychiatric provider if you have one, a healthcare professional, or someone in your core group of contacts. You want to talk to someone who will listen to you without judgment or criticism. You might start by saying, "I don't know but I've been feeling quite low lately. Do you have any suggestions for me?" If you have thoughts of ending your life, I highly recommend calling 911 or another crisis or emergency line in your locality as a matter of urgency. Believe it or not, your life is more valuable than you think. God wants you alive more than you think. Believe it or not, your life will go on beyond the roadblock that you see right now. Believe it or not, this one, too, shall pass—I promise you! Above all, I know that God has a special plan for your life that is yet to unfold. Remember the popular saying, "A problem shared is a problem halved."

Sometimes when you are in crisis, people in your life will provide support naturally. However, you don't want to wait until you're in crisis to receive this support. You can begin to develop relationships with your contacts that will grow them into your support system in case you get into a crisis situation. How do you develop more meaningful relationships with your contacts? You must be intentional about it. You cannot leave this to chance. Relationships are developed through regular communication and beneficial interactions. Some of the most effective tools for developing relationships are periodic face-to-face small talk, a quick call, or text message, such as, "How're you doing today?" "What's going on with you?" "I hope everything is fine with you." "You have a blessed day."

Practice Kindness, Reach out to Others

Another powerful tool for developing relationships that will turn your contacts into your support system is reaching out to help others. I know you might be thinking, "Given the state that I am in, what do I have to give to others?" You would be surprised to note that simple gestures of reaching out to show concern, offer a non-judgmental listening ear, or actually help others can bring so much satisfaction and emotional healing into your life. It is the same principle in volunteering to support various causes in your local area, donating to charity, and offering your gifts and expertise to others in some way. When you take the challenge, I need to warn you that it will appear strange.

It may appear strange because traditionally, our society expects that when a person depressed or ill, that person would be on the receiving end of acts of kindness, not on the giving end. Well, I throw you a challenge—receive all the help that is available to you but gather the courage and move over to the giving end. You may be pleasantly surprised that there is more healing and fulfilment on the giving end. Many people do not take advantage of this, but there is so much healing and fulfillment on the giving end of relationships. It is sad to note that only a few people are on the giving end of relationships nowadays. Most people seem to be enjoying the receiving end, and they are reluctant to move over. Dare to move over to the giving end, and you will taste healing like never before.

Find a Support Group

In many communities, there are support groups for just about anything that you may be going through. The website 211.org hosts several community resources while another website Meetup.com provides opportunities for people with various interests to network and interact with others in similar situations. Fellowshipping regularly with church groups or participating in depression or anxiety support groups in your neighborhood are a key opportunity for mutual support and the healing that comes with it. You may consider enrolling in programs at the Young Men's Christian Association (YMCA) or the Young Women Christian Association (YWMA). Your local library or hospital may have more information on support groups or opportunities for social connection.

Three Levels of Relationship

According to Dr. Mensa Otabil, in your efforts to become socially connected, it is important to include three groups of people in your life—people ahead of you, people at your level, and people behind you. Those who are ahead of you may include people who suffered with depression but are no longer depressed or those who have experience helping others who are depressed. This group of people will make deposits into your life that will speed up your healing process. The second group are those who are currently at your level, actively going through what you are going through. These are people that you share with and who make you understand that your situation is not abnormal. As explored earlier, the third group of people you might want to connect with are those who are behind you in your journey to lasting healing from depression. Believe it or not, there are millions of people whose situation is worse than yours. These are people whose lives you make deposits into. The more often you empty your barrel, the more you will be replenished and the fresher the contents will be.

Chapter 8

The Professional Dimension

"Coming together is a beginning. Keeping together is progress. Working together is success."
– Henry Ford

I n this chapter, I am going to address the role that psychiatric and psychological professionals can play in your healing process. Just like a headache, depression comes in various forms and with various levels of severity depending on its history, duration, and presenting symptoms. Mild to moderate depression may respond to any combination of non-pharmacological interventions, meaning that you may get well without the need to take medications. Even then, several questions arise: How do you know that what you are going through is depression and no other illness? Several conditions may show up with many of the same symptoms as depression. Examples of such illnesses are hypothyroidism, hormonal imbalances especially among women, some forms of cancer, side effects of some medications, alcohol abuse, and cannabis dependence. It takes a thorough examination by medically trained psychiatric professional to determine the difference.

Psychiatric Professionals

Let me provide a short overview of the differences among the various mental health healing professionals in the United States. Psychiatrists are medical doctors who also completed residency training in psychiatry. They are licensed to prescribe medications and provide psychotherapy, and they use the designation MD or DO after their names. Psychologists hold Ph.D. degrees and are licensed to provide therapy and conduct specialized testing. They do not typically prescribe medications, though a few states have started granting prescriptive privileges to psychologists as well.

Psychiatric and mental health nurse practitioners (PMHNPs) are first registered nurses who went on and obtained advanced degrees, either master's degrees or doctoral degrees in psychiatric nursing and are licensed to prescribe medications and provide psychotherapy as well. Similarly, physician assistants (PAs) hold master's degrees and are licensed to prescribe medications and provide therapy. Social workers typically hold master's degrees and may be licensed to provide psychotherapy but do not prescribe medications. Other clinical professionals that you may encounter in this field include registered nurses, licensed professional nurses, certified nursing assistants, behavioral health technicians, medical assistants, and peer support specialists.

Emergency Departments

As you can see, there are several experts and treatment settings in the mental health field. Obviously, when the symptoms of depression are severe, it is wise to seek expert help as soon as possible in order to prevent adverse outcomes, as every passing day could mean that you're getting a situation where a lengthy hospitalization and/or treatment may become necessary.

If you call an emergency line for help, an emergency response team may be dispatched to help you. In some communities, you may can call a mental health crisis line, where a crisis worker will speak with you over the phone and walk you through what you need to do to maintain safety. If it happens that you are taken to the emergency department of a hospital, various assessments will be done by the emergency department doctor, who may then order a psychiatry consult if he thinks this is necessary. If you are taken to a mental health crisis center, a psychiatric evaluation will be done, initial treatment will be given, and a decision will be made whether it is important to continue with inpatient psychiatric hospital admission or not.

Crisis Response Centers

Typically, both emergency departments and crisis centers provide essential emergency care for anyone whose life is in danger or who is a threat to the safety of others. The difference between the two is that mental health crisis centers are usually staffed with specialized psychiatric providers while emergency departments may or may not have specialized psychiatric providers.

A few nights a week, I see patients at a psychiatric crisis center. This center is staffed with psychiatrists, nurse practitioners, physician assistants, psychiatric nurses, crisis workers, behavioral health technicians, and peer-review specialists who provide a range of crisis psychiatric interventions to help stabilize our patients in about twenty-four hours.

It is phenomenal to see the turnaround from the initial presentation of our patients to how they present at the time of discharge. This difference is often like night and day. After people are discharged from the crisis center or hospital, they typically are asked to follow up with an outpatient psychiatric provider, who establishes ongoing mental health care with the aim of restoring the individual to his or her original emotional state and level of functioning. Most outpatient psychiatric providers (psychiatrist or psychiatric nurse practitioner) establish a therapeutic relationship with the individual and his/her family or significant others in order to make recommendations and treatment decisions from an informed perspective.

Outpatient Psychiatric Services

In the case of depression that is non-life-threatening, it is important that you make an appointment to see a psychiatrist or a psychiatric nurse practitioner for a comprehensive psychiatric evaluation and treatment recommendations including medication considerations. Alternatively, you may see a psychologist or a psychotherapist for a clinical evaluation and treatment recommendations without medication options. It is important to call ahead of time and schedule an appointment, bring with you a picture identification card, a list of medications that you're currently taking, and a means of payment for your services—insurance card or other means of payment.

After your initial encounter, you may be scheduled to follow-up at a later time. Between appointments, it may be helpful if you could maintain a journal of your mood daily by writing down how you're feeling. Bring this journal with you to your next appointment to help your provider understand the nature of your problem better. There are also cellphone apps for tracking your mood and you may be able to share the results with your provider at/before your follow-up meetings.

The Psychiatric Evaluation

A typical comprehensive psychiatric evaluation will involve the assessment of your height and weight, your vital signs (such as blood pressure, heart rate, and respiratory rate), and an interview section that covers several areas. Obviously, the provider would like to understand why you are seeking help at this time, what symptoms you are experiencing and for how long, how severe they are, and what worsens or what lessens your symptoms. This is what we call your chief complaint and history of present illness. However, the provider is not only interested in what is going on now. We are also interested in any aspects of your history that are pertinent to your current presentation. We may start with basic demographical information such as your name, your age, address, contact phone, preferred languages, your allergies to medications (if any), and your emergency contact person.

Next, the provider would like to understand your life's journey by asking questions about your past psychiatric history. This includes your past psychiatric diagnoses, previous psychiatric providers, medications that you took in the past and whether they were effective or not, if you have had any mental health hospitalization, or history of self-harm or suicide attempts. We also like to know if you have or had any medical or physical health conditions or surgeries and other health care providers that you're currently working with.

Other areas of interest in a psychiatric evaluation may include any mental health or substance abuse problems in your immediate family, your childhood experience, any history of physical, emotional or sexual abuse or trauma that you might have suffered, your social history including marital status and family composition/structure, social connections, developmental history including any history of delays in meeting developmental milestones, your highest educational level, occupation, and any major legal history that you have. Finally, we conduct a substance abuse history so we can understand what addictive substances you currently use or have used in the past and to what extent. Some of the substances that we may be interested in are coffee, tobacco, alcohol, street drugs such as cocaine, heroin, and methamphetamine, and prescription medications as well. Your provider may also ask questions regarding other addictions, such as gambling.

Beyond the above, you may be asked to complete a few questionnaires that would be analyzed and interpreted by your provider. You may also be asked to complete other tasks to help the provider to assess your mental status. Comprehensive labs and a urine drug test may be ordered to include complete blood count, comprehensive metabolic profile, lipid profile, thyroid level, and HbA1c (which measures your risk of becoming diabetic). With your permission, your family and friends, who know you well, may be contacted for further information about the course and nature of your illness from their perspective. This process is typical for psychiatrists and psychiatric nurse practitioners. The process will be different if you saw a master's level psychotherapist, a psychologist, or a pastoral mental health counselor.

Additional Assessments

In my practice, in addition to the above, I conduct a spiritual assessment to understand your belief system, your values, a self-efficacy assessment that includes your life's mission, a detailed social assessment, and an assessment of your nutritional habits and physical exercise practices. After this process, I would assign a working diagnosis and negotiate a treatment plan with you including tasks that we will complete together and homework tasks that you will complete on your own for discussion at our future meetings. I usually ask for your consent/agreement and commitment to the plan before proceeding with treatment.

Comorbid Substance Addiction

If you happen to have a problem with substance addiction, it may be important to seek treatment for this first or alongside your depression treatment. It is often hard to tell which came first—substance addiction or depression. This is because, on one hand when people are depressed, they are more prone to abusing substances, and on the other hand, people with substance abuse problems are at a higher risk of becoming depressed. For moderate to severe substance abuse, long-term residential rehabilitation or intensive outpatient programs come recommended. Whatever the case, treating depression without treating comorbid substance addiction is not only unwise but will not provide the desired results.

Primary Care Providers

Note that, owing to the limited number of mental health professionals in most parts of the world in relation to the population, you may receive treatment for depression from a primary care professional. This is totally appropriate. Primary care professionals include internal medicine doctors and family nurse practitioners, who are also trained to identify and provide basic psychiatry services. They may do a referral to a psychiatric specialist if your treatment becomes more complex or they believe that you need specialized attention.

Psychotherapy

To conclude this chapter, I would like to explore the role of psychotherapy and some therapy modalities that may be helpful to you in your treatment. Psychotherapy (or *therapy* for short) may be described as the deliberate use of talk and psychological techniques to help alleviate suffering or manage mental, emotional, or substance abuse disorders. The current data on the effectiveness of psychotherapy indicates that about seventy-five per cent of individuals who participate in therapy have derived at least some benefit from it.[25] Therapy sessions are typically held anywhere from once weekly or once every other week for a duration of thirty to fifty minutes.

Psychotherapy Modalities

There are many forms of psychotherapy, including cognitive behavioral therapy, dialectical behavior therapy, mindfulness, and eye movement desensitization and reprocessing (EMDR). Each therapy modality lends itself to conditions that they are best suited for.

Cognitive Behavioral Therapy (CBT): CBT is the most common psychotherapy approach for depression and anxiety. It is a structured approach to helping recognize unhealthy thought and behavior patterns that you might have and replace them with healthier alternatives. CBT helps to define what is going on in your life and your thoughts and beliefs about what is going on, and it helps you to see complex situations in clearer and more objective ways. It also equips you with psychological and lifestyle tools that you can utilize in your healing process.

In my practice, I frequently utilize both traditional CBT and a unique type of CBT called Christian Cognitive Behavioral Therapy (CCBT). CCBT is the use of Christ-centered Bible-based tools and resources to solve mental health and emotional problems. It is like harnessing the best of the worlds of science and faith.

Dialectical Behavioral Therapy (DBT): This is a therapy modality used with individuals who are chronically self-harming and those who have been diagnosed with borderline personality disorder. The aim is to reduce self-injurious behaviors and to help the individual to improve his/her interpersonal relationships.

Eye Movement Desensitization and Reprocessing (EMDR): This is a psychotherapy modality used to relieve the suffering that results from traumatic memories.

Each therapy modality requires specialized qualifications and training on the part of the therapist in order to implement it properly. Therapy may be offered in an individual or group setting depending on the setting and the agreement between you and your therapist. I believe you appreciate the vast amount of professional resources available in the psychiatric and psychological fields to help you navigate through the dark emotional clouds that surround you. You definitely don't have to do this alone, my friend!

Chapter 9

Yes, You Have Options!

*"If you don't jump, you won't swim.
If you don't swim, you won't float."*

Congratulations for reading this far! You have just demonstrated that you have what it takes to start walking out of the dark place. In this chapter, I will show you some of the obstacles that will confront you on your way to recovering from depression. The first obstacle is doubt—doubt in God's ability to heal you, doubt in your ability to heal, and doubt in the process of your healing. Once you remember that it does not cost anything to believe, you will begin to unleash your faith at the mountain that stands before you. Dare to believe! You must heal, and you will heal! Think about your unfulfilled dreams! You wish you were actively involved in your family's activities. You wish you were delivering on your purpose. Has it ever struck you that the world is eagerly waiting for what you are carrying? How about this?—The next generation is waiting in line for you to deliver on your part of the bargain. You can't drop the ball. No! Not at this time!

The Obstacle of Inaction

That's not all. You will encounter the obstacle of inaction. Depression literally holds you down and keeps you from taking action. I call it the inertia factor. Inertia is the tendency to resist change and maintain the status quo. In life, there are many people who truly want to make progress but are seriously idle. They are strategically positioning themselves to act someday. Believe me—It is easier to remain where you have been than to initiate action towards where you could be. Your dream of living a vibrant, productive, and depression-free life will only happen when you put wheels to your dreams.

In all my years of working with people who have walked the journey of recovery, one thing is clear: Lasting cure does require deliberate effort on the part of the person that is seeking to heal. You have heard the saying that faith without works is dead (James 2:25). There was a man at the pool of Bethesda, who wanted to be healed. You can find his story in John 5:1-15 in the Bible. From time to time, an angel would come and stir the water and whoever stepped into the water first would be healed. This gentleman had been ill for thirty-eight years. He was only one step away from being healed, but his healing had remained a dream because he was waiting—yes, he was waiting for so long as "there was no one" to help him step into the water.

Nothing Ventured, Nothing Gained

Similarly, you can also decide to do nothing about your situation. I hope this is not the case for anyone, including you. This is because if you ever fell in this category you will not merely remain where you are. You have heard it said, "nothing ventured, nothing gained." While that may be true in some situations, in the case of untreated depression, the truth is that when nothing is ventured, everything is lost. Untreated depression usually becomes worse over time. Moderate symptoms will become severe. Severe symptoms usually become strongholds that can literally stop you from living. My prayer is that you don't fall in this category. No! This is not you, and it is not an option. Let's move on to your actual options.

In the story of the man at the pool, it would interest you to note that the man did not heal just because Jesus showed up. Also, Jesus did not just heal him just because He could. There is a God-part and a man-part in every miracle. When Jesus showed up at the pool, he first demanded faith from the man by asking him if he wanted to get well. Next, Jesus demanded action! There is no victory without a battle. You will not win if you don't fight. Get over your resistance to act and get moving towards your goal of a depression-free life. But—wait a minute!

The Illusion of Quick Solutions

Another obstacle is the search for quick solutions. In these days of drive-throughs and microwaves, quick fixes are a real threat to true, sustained, and authentic healing. I wish there was a quick fix to achieving a lasting cure from depression! I wish that healing from depression was a short, one-hundred-meter dash! But it is not. Your approach must not be deliberate only but consistent. The fact that something is hard to do does not mean that it is impossible. Just like every proven system, the AHPD will only work for you when you work it. You are at a critical crossroad in your transformation process. You acquired a vast amount of information regarding evidence-based approaches to healing from depression. Now, let's look at the true options that are available to you.

Do It Yourself

You can hit the ground running and implement some of the things you learned from this book on your own. You must be proud of yourself if you are in this group. You can lay out the various aspects of the AHPD, prepare an individualized recovery program for yourself, and start your journey to recovery. You will need to start from the what is easiest for you to do first or what is fully within your control and move on from there. Remember to reward yourself for every victory won. You don't have to wait until you feel better before you reward yourself. Just connecting socially or just implementing a thirty-minute, every other day workout program is enough to start rewarding yourself. Be careful not to reward yourself with unhealthy treats that would wipe out the gains you have already made. This option is important because you will always have to do a lot by yourself even if you went with the other options that we will talk about ahead. I can say that just by starting, you are half-way through.

One challenge with this approach is that you will be doing this alone. However, this process is going to require a great deal of effort from you. To enhance your chances of success, you can implement the process together with a partner who shares your interests and is willing to walk the journey with you. Appoint a person who you would be accountable to and empower this person to hold you responsible to what you have committed to doing. Another challenge is that you may not have the expertise required for some components of the AHPD, such as clinical training and spiritual insight. That is not to say that you will be unsuccessful implementing the process by yourself. With God, nothing shall be impossible!

Work with a Professional

Third, you can reach out for professional help. You may call up a psychiatric provider, make an appointment, collaborate with this person to draw up an action plan, and stick to the plan for a reasonable period of time. Again, do not expect overnight results and do not quit because you are not getting results; modify the plan and keep going! With your current level of insight, you probably know what kind of professional will be most appropriate for you. People who choose this option are more likely to achieve results than those who attempt to do it alone. This is based on the premise that implementing the interventions shared in this book will help you heal but you may never get around to it by yourself. This is why you are going to need someone to work with you.

The challenge here is that each provider is different in what they believe and what they are willing to incorporate into their treatment process. Your provider may believe in medications but not supplements. Your provider may believe in therapy but not spirituality. Your provider may believe in all the aspects of the AHPD, but he or she may not be able to incorporate all the aspects into his/her practice as most practices are designed to provide only one aspect of the AHPD. Most practices provide medication management services and maybe therapy but not faith interventions or opportunities for social connection. Most workplaces do not even allow the mention of faith practices in their work with clients.

Reach out to Me!

The final option available to you is that you may want to reach out to me for help. I know you're thinking, "Really?" My answer is, "Why not?" Of course, you will need to consult with me or one of my team members to ensure that we can work together. I offer a free initial consultation by phone during which I am glad to learn about you and what you are trying to accomplish. It is important for me that I understand your journey up until now and what you are looking to accomplish. I value teamwork, flexibility, and creativity, but once we develop a collaborative plan, I usually ask that we stick to it until we get results. The goal is for you to have total and lasting cure from depression and accomplish your mission on earth.

Over the past several years, I have worked with several individuals in community health, outpatient, inpatient, crisis, and church settings who had great success overcoming depression. Some of my clients have left feedback for me, which you might find helpful.[26] Even more exciting, I am currently launching a unique Christian integrative psychiatric program where I can teach the contents of this book, coach individuals and groups, and literally join and walk with my clients on their unforgettable journeys out of the darkness of depression into the light of their dreams come true. This is what I am called to do. I am a channel of hope!

Chapter 10
Concluding Thoughts

"Knowing is not enough; we must apply.
Willing is not enough; we must do."
– Johann Wolfgang von Goethe

L et's do a quick recap of what we covered in this volume. I want to make sure that you do not lose focus on the essential things to note from this book. First, in Chapter One, we explored your situation. You have found yourself in a less than desirable place in life. You just happen to be where you are. You did not ask for it and I bet you feel that you do not deserve to be in this emotional hole. You are depressed, and life is a chore. You sometimes wish it would all be over.

In Chapter Two, we took a walk along the path of my life. My journey has been full of discoveries. It appears as if all along life has been preparing us to be right here, working together toward the common goal of bringing you to where you need to be—cured of depression! You deserve to be permanently healed and to enjoy a fulfilling life here on earth and beyond.

In order to accomplish this desire, in Chapter Three, we explored the one tool that has been tested, tried, and proven to bring lasting healing from depression—the AHPD. You understood that the current piecemeal approaches to treating depression do not always work and that there is a need for a truly holistic, comprehensive, and long-term approach. As you can see, the AHPD is more of a long-term lifestyle modification process than a quick-fix solution to depression. While some people may have rapid results, anyone who is looking for a quick fix will soon become disappointed along the way.

Starting from Chapter Four, we explored the AHPD domains in more detail. We expounded on the self-efficacy domain. I hope you appreciate the leading role that you play in the process of your healing. If there is one thing you should take away from this chapter, you should understand that your healing is more likely to occur when you take on a leading role in the process. You should understand that the discovery, development, and deployment of your purpose in life are a core component of lasting healing from depression. We also talked about the power of your mind in helping produce your desired outcome in life.

In Chapter Five, we dove into the world of biochemistry, where we understood that there is often an underlying chemical imbalance involved in depression. If you are going to achieve lasting healing from depression, this imbalance must be corrected. The chemical imbalance can be corrected through several ways, including taking antidepressant medications, supplements, exercising regularly, sleeping adequately, eating healthy, and engaging in relaxation techniques.

In Chapter Six, we delved into the spiritual world. I hope you appreciate the fact that man is spirit with a soul and lives in a body. How connected you are to your source is important in your healing process. In fact, emotional healing without concomitant spiritual healing is an effort in futility. Closely reflect on this and open your spirit for the deep-seated healing that will bring overall healing to you like never before. The arms of the Lord are wide open. He is longing to reconnect with you and take you on His wings.

Chapter Seven was an exploration of social connectedness. We learned that the people in our lives can be as good as medicine. We only need to change the way we see them, deliberately cultivate our relationships, and leverage them to our advantage. You have a wealth of gold in the people around you. Do not ignore this source of healing.

We concluded the AHPD dimensions in Chapter Eight by addressing the need for you to work with the experts in the field of psychiatry and psychology and beyond. There is high value in working with the right professionals. You need to know who is out there and who to call for what you're looking for.

I hope you see that the AHPD is not a quick-fix method for treating depression that only produces short-term results. The AHPD aims to enhance your entire lifestyle. Beyond healing from depression, the AHPD is meant to make you a better person, bring out the best in you, and secure you an eternal destiny, hope for the future, and confidence for today.

After all the components of the AHPD were discussed, we explored the next steps that are available to you in Chapter Nine. You can choose to do nothing, which should not be an option. You can embark on a solo journey with a determination to overcome your depression, which is difficult but not impossible. You can work with other professionals, which is recommended if you can find professionals who also believe in the AHPD. Ultimately, you may reach out to work with me. As much as I am able, I would like to be part of your journey to recovery from depression or provide you with further resources to aid you in your journey.

Intentionality

As mentioned earlier, the AHPD will only work when you work it. Modern society is so busy that you will have multiple commitments competing for the same spots in your daily routine. For this reason, anything that is left to chance will most likely not get done. This is where intentionality comes in. This is why the famous German author, Goethe, wrote, "Knowing is not enough; we must apply. Willing is not enough; we must do." One way to ensure that you can move from knowledge to implementation is to write down every intended activity on your daily schedule. In my life, I have come to realize that if it is not on the schedule, it may not get done. Another technique is to schedule activities with someone else (the buddy system). This works for physical exercise and church attendance. The idea behind the buddy system is that your buddy may be motivated to act and literally pull you along, even if you are not motivated at the time.

Daily Routine

I am confident that you can overcome depression. Yes! Your life can take on a new meaning! You can live a fulfilled life here on earth and you can look forward to a glorious life after death as well. What a double win! This, however, will take a habitual approach to accomplish, not short-term random or casual efforts. Aristotle was quoted as saying, "We are what we repeatedly do. Excellence, therefore, is not an act, but a habit." To this end, I have included below suggestions for a daily routine. Consider integrating as much of it as possible into your daily life and see the results for yourself.

Suggested Activities for
Total Healing from Depression

Activity	Corresponding AHPD Dimension
1. Offer thanks to God first thing in the morning.	Spiritual dimension
2. Read a portion of the Bible and go over your affirmations in the morning. Say the following every morning: I. "This is the day the Lord has made; I will rejoice and be glad in it" (Psalm 118:24, modified by author). II. In Christ Jesus, I am more than a conqueror!	Spiritual dimension
3. Read out your life's mission. You had placed it on the wall, remember? Take a little step towards your mission by acting on your daily goals from the night before.	Self-efficacy dimension
4. Take your medications, if prescribed. Drink a tall glass of water with your medications.	Biochemical dimension

5. Meet with the professionals you are working with (if scheduled).	Professional dimension
6. "Eat breakfast like a king, lunch like a prince, and dinner like a pauper."	Biochemical dimension
7. Workout at least thirty minutes a day.	Biochemical dimension
8. Engage in meaningful social contact with others (playing a sport, holding hands, doing a project, praying together, studying the Bible together, et cetera).	Social dimension
9. Practice gratitude, joy, positive coping, and kindness. Do something kind for someone today.	Self-efficacy dimension and spiritual dimension
10. Practice bedtime meditation. Write your goals for the next day. Maintain a regular bedtime schedule.	Spiritual dimension and biochemical dimension

"Make time for rest but… No matter how you feel… Get up, dress up, show up, and never give up!"
–Anonymous

My wish for you!

My first wish for you is that you will achieve lasting, possibly permanent, recovery from depression. I wish that you remain open-minded enough that you will benefit from Western medications, complementary therapies, and working with professionals in the field of psychiatry, psychology, and Christian faith interventions. I hope you will be successful in making a psychological shift from a defeatist mindset to that of a truly liberated individual. I wish that you will be successful in regularizing your sleep and appetite and stay energized. I want you to truly enjoy your relationships, improve your work productivity, and love what you do. Above all, I wish that you will derive eternal benefits from the darkest moments of your life.

There will be no better time than now to tackle your depression. If it must be done, then it must be done NOW, and if it must be done, then it must be done WELL. I pray that you will have a renewed hope in your ability to find true and lasting joy. One thing I know is that there is hope for your future (Jeremiah 29:11). I pray that you will have a renewed sense of purpose and become more motivated and energized to pursue your purpose while enjoying the peace of God in the process. May a switch turn on in your soul and may the light of God shine through your darkness. Develop a new confidence in God's ability to heal you and restore joy to you.

A Call to Action

Determine to live the rest of your life with Jesus Christ as your Lord and Master, the church and spiritual practices as your source of nourishment, friends and family as stakeholders, and other humans as your mission field. May you find and develop healthy relationships with professionals in various fields. I hope that your world has expanded, and you will find value in leveraging multiple resources for lasting healing. Do not leave anything on the table in your healing process. Your life and destiny are at stake.

I speak total and permanent healing into your life. Receive lasting joy here on earth and find rest with our Maker in heaven. I desire to meet you in heaven, running toward me with a scream, saying, "Thank you for investing in my life! I am here because of you!" Ultimate significance in life is when you hear God say to you, "Well done, good and faithful servant; you were faithful over a few things, I will make you ruler over many things. Enter into the joy of your lord" (Matthew 25:23). Shalom! Peace and grace to you!

Acknowledgments

S ir Isaac Newton is quoted as saying, "If I have seen further, it is by standing on the shoulders of giants." That's true for me as I have stood on so many shoulders that I have lost count. I am first grateful to God because if it had not been for Him on my side, I have no idea where I would be. I am forever grateful to my wife and life-partner, Esenam, whose relentless encouragement, team spirit, and sacrifices have brought me this far. To our children, Elsie, Ellis, and Elton, thank you for lending me to the world.

My true heroes are my parents, Nathaniel Kwakuyi and Gladys Gletsu, and my nine siblings, all of whom have been used by God in significant ways to nurture and mold me into such a fine gentleman (Ha!). For this book and the next phase of my career, I am thankful for Dr. Angela Lauria, my business coach, Cory Hott, Ora North, and Trevor McCray, my editors, and the entire Author Incubator team for helping me launch a movement of global proportions. Many thanks to David Hancock and the Morgan James Publishing team for helping me bring this book to print.

I am a product of the following mentors, whom God has placed at strategic points in my life to help bring out the best in me: Dr. Mensa Otabil (Founder and General Overseer of the International Central Gospel Church, ICGC), the late Dr. Myles Munroe, Dr. Robin Ross of COPE Community Services, Pastor Rick Warren of the Saddleback Church, Bishop Dag Heward-Mills of Lighthouse Chapel International, Ms. Mary Lou Graham, Nurse Practitioner in New Britain, Connecticut, Mr. Albert Wilson of Wilson Consortium (Ghana), and Mr. Dan Acquaye of ASNAPP (Ghana).

I thank my loving pastors and spiritual fathers for their sacrifice, guidance, and insight: Pastor Fred Akpai (Colorado), Rev. Nat Akyeampong (New York), Rev. Sampson Yeboah (Connecticut), Rev. Dr. Frank Opoku-Amoako (Virginia), Rev. Emmanuel Owusu-Kyereko (Georgia), Rev. Rick Donkor (California), Pastor Peter Dzandza (New York), Pastor Glenn Bone (Texas), and Pastor Paul Boakye-Dattey (Connecticut). This list cannot end without a special mention of Pastor Theodore Dzeble (Ghana) and my brother Ernest Kwakuyi (Ghana), who coached me, read over the manuscript, and provided valuable feedback, as well as my sister Perfect Kwakuyi (Virginia) and my cousin Dr. Janet Dzator (Australia), who provided much guidance along the way.

Finally, I am forever grateful to the leadership and members of my church family at ICGC Impact Chapel in Tucson, Arizona (I love you lots!), my numerous friends and partners, notably, Jeff Dixon, psychotherapist and Gloria Ramos, who work with me at the Tucson Treatment Center, and my coworkers at the Crisis Response Center. You're my world!

References

1   World Health Organization (WHO). 2013. Mental
    Health Action Plan 2013-2030, Geneva, Switzerland

2   The 2018 World Health Organization Fact Sheet on
    Depression. Retrieved from https://www.who.int/news-
    room/fact-sheets/detail/depression

3   The National Institute of Mental Health 2017 Report on
    Major Depression. Retrieved from https://www.nimh.nih.
    gov/health/statistics/major-depression.shtml

4   Matthew 17:15-18 (NKJV). Retrieved from https://
    www.biblegateway.com/passage/?search=Mat-
    thew+17%3A15-18&version=NKJV

5   Cuijpers, Pim; Sijbrandij, Marit; Koole, Sander L; Anders-
    son, Gerhard; Beekman, Aartjan T; et al. World psychiatry :
    official journal of the World Psychiatric Association (WPA)
    Vol. 12, Iss. 2, (June 2013): 137-148. And Kolovos,

Spyros; van Tulder, Maurits W; Cuijpers, Pim; Prigent, Amélie; Chevreul, Karine; et al.Journal of affective disorders Vol. 210, (March 1, 2017): 72-81.

6   Engel, G.L. The need for a new medical model: A challenge for biomedicine. Science 1977, 196, 129–136. [CrossRef] [PubMed] and Engel, G.L. The biopsychosocial model and the education of health professionals. Ann. N. Y. Acad. Sci. 1978, 310, 169–187. [CrossRef] [PubMed]

7   Bandura, Albert (1982). "Self-efficacy mechanism in human agency". American Psychologist. 37 (2): 122–147. doi:10.1037/0003-066X.37.2.122.

8   Sadock, Benjamin J., Virginia A. Sadock, and Pedro Ruiz. Kaplan & Sadock's Synopsis of Psychiatry: Behavioral Sciences/clinical Psychiatry. Tenth edition, Pages 529-532. Philadelphia: Wolters Kluwer, 2007.

9   Hasler, Gregor. "Pathophysiology of depression: do we have any solid evidence of interest to clinicians?" World psychiatry: official journal of the World Psychiatric Association (WPA) vol. 9,3 (2010): 155-61.

10   https://www.verywellmind.com/albert-bandura-biography-1925-2795537

11   https://pdfs.semanticscholar.org/8bee/c556fe7a650120544a99e9e063eb8fcd987b.pdf

12   Courtesy: Doris Hill, MSW

13   Greenberg, P. E., Fournier, A. A., Sisitsky, T., Pike, C. T., & Kessler, R. C. (2015). The economic burden of adults with major depressive disorder in the United States (2005 and 2010). Journal of Clinical Psychiatry, 76, 155–162. doi: 10.4088/JCP.14m09298

14 Slavich, George M, and Michael R Irwin. "From stress to inflammation and major depressive disorder: a social signal transduction theory of depression." Psychological bulletin vol. 140,3 (2014): 774-815. doi:10.1037/a0035302

15 https://dashdiet.org/mediterranean-diet.html

16 https://www.rush.edu/news/press-releases/dash-style-diet-associated-reduced-risk-depression

17 https://www.ncbi.nlm.nih.gov/pmc/articles/PMC5430071/#B42

18 https://www.ncbi.nlm.nih.gov/pmc/articles/PMC5430071/#B42

19 Courtesy: Comfort Impraim, FNP-BC, MSN

20 https://www.thelancet.com/journals/lancet/article/PIIS0140-6736(17)32802-7/fulltext

21 Sadock, Benjamin J., Virginia A. Sadock, and Pedro Ruiz. Kaplan & Sadock's Synopsis of Psychiatry: Behavioral Sciences/clinical Psychiatry. Tenth edition, Pages 529-532. Philadelphia: Wolters Kluwer, 2007.

22 Ng, Qin Xiang, Nandini Venkatanarayanan, and Collin Yih Xian Ho. "Clinical use of Hypericum Perforatum (St John's Wort) in Depression: A Meta-Analysis." Journal of Affective Disorders 210, (2017): 211-221.

23 https://hymnary.org/text/when_upon_lifes_billows_you_are_tempest

24 Taylor, Harry Owen, Robert Joseph Taylor, Ann W. Nguyen, and Linda Chatters. "Social Isolation, Depression, and Psychological Distress Among Older Adults." Journal of Aging and Health 30, no. 2 (February 2018): 229–46. doi:10.1177/0898264316673511. And Sanders, Christo-

pher E., et al. "The Relationship of Internet use to Depression and Social Isolation among Adolescents." Adolescence 35.138 (2000): 237-42. ProQuest. Web. 6 May 2019.

25   American Psychological Association. Understanding psychotherapy and how it works. 2016. http://www.apa.org/helpcenter/understanding-psychotherapy.aspx

26   www.healthgrades.com/providers/joy-kwakuyi-xymjhdb

Thank You!

I am grateful that you have read *The Ultimate Cure for Depression?* This is the beginning of greater things to come in your life. According to Psalm 30:5, "Weeping may endure for a night, but joy comes in the morning." My prayer for you is that you will find lasting joy and fulfillment in your life.

However, the sweetness of the pudding is in the eating. You will only benefit from the material in this book if you implement the best-practices that I discussed. Please do not neglect to share this book with a loved one. You will be starting a healing revolution around the world.

I would love to hear about the results you are getting. I would also like to be part of your journey to recovery from depression. Feel free to contact me via:

My website: www.tucsontreatment.com

My email: drjoy@tucsontreatment.com

My Facebook page:

https://www.facebook.com/Tucson-Treatment-Center-Inc-1750944985233761/

My LinkedIn page:

https://www.linkedin.com/in/joy-kwakuyi-dnp-pmhnp-5bb00115/

My YouTube page:

https://www.youtube.com/channel/UCEudkJGVlqdQ2zXAOgiXORA? view_as=subscriber

Free Video Class

As my appreciation to you for reading this book, I am offering you a FREE gift. I will make available to you a free video class on, "The Authentic Healing Process for Depression" at the videos section of my website (www.tucsontreatment.com). This is a class that I prepared for my coaching clients. It contains clear and concise steps to achieving total and lasting healing from depression. Feel free to watch this video and provide me with feedback via email. God Bless You!

About the Author

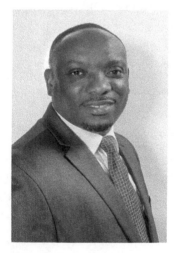

Dr. Joy Kwakuyi is a respected integrative psychiatric nurse practitioner, pastor, and life coach, who helps leaders and professionals to find total and lasting relief from depression and anxiety. He is the owner and director of the Tucson Treatment Center (www.tucsontreatment.com), where he works with politicians, business and non-profit executives, lawyers, pastors, and healthcare professionals, and speaks to various audiences with the goal of optimizing their psychosocial functioning and finding fulfillment in life. In his work, he leverages and advocates integrative psychiatric and Christian interventions based on his Authentic Healing Process for Depression (AHPD) treatment process. He also sits on the medical executive committee and peer review committee at Connections Health Solutions.

Dr. Kwakuyi holds a Doctor of Nursing Practice degree and a Master of Science degree from the University of South Alabama, a bachelor's degree and a post baccalaureate certificate in nursing from the University of Connecticut, a master's degree from the University of London, and a bachelor's degree from the Kwame Nkrumah University of Science and Technology in Ghana. He has about fifteen years of experience working in various sectors, with thirty years of Christian ministry experience in Africa, Europe, and the U.S.A.

Dr. Kwakuyi spends his life providing hope and healing to the emotionally hurting. With the help of his wife and friends, he started and pastors the International Central Gospel Church (ICGC) Impact Chapel in Tucson (www.impactchapel.org). Dr. Kwakuyi and his wife, Esenam, live in Tucson with their three children, Elsie, Ellis, and Elton.